ADVANCE PRAISE FOR *TWIN SET*

"*Twin Set* is a saving grace. Equal parts friend, therapist, and teacher, the book provides a realistic—and funny!—snapshot into what really goes on in the homes and minds of moms of multiples. Nonjudgmental, genuine, and helpful, this book is a drop of water to the desert of multiples books currently out there."

—Amy Newman, associate publisher, *Cookie* (and mother of twins)

"If a book can be called a friend, then *Twin Set* fills the role seamlessly. It is the ideal companion for any new or expecting mommy of multiples and will have you parenting with confidence, heart, and style."

—Samantha Ettus, creator of *The Experts' Guide to the Baby Years*

"I wish I'd had this book with my twins . . . the advice is practical and helpful, but most of all, knowing that there are other moms out there who get what it's like to have twins is a huge comfort."

—Jane Seymour, actress and mother of twins

"*Twin Set* is a great resource and a quick read. It covers everything a new twin parent will need to know in an organized and quick manner! The section on preemies is crucial for those parents who need the extra words of wisdom to care for their fragile babies."

—Elizabeth S. Klein, president, The Tiny Miracles Foundation

"It was about time for a modern, thorough, and HONEST twin guide. I wish I had *Twin Set* a year ago, when my twin guys were born."

—Patty Onderko, senior editor at *Babytalk* magazine (and mother of twins)

"*Twin Set* is a terrific book; I especially like the balanced views the authors offer. Their pro-and-con approach gives new parents the power to choose what's best for their own children. *Twin Set* is Big Picture parenting—plus all the latest details—written with a positive attitude and just enough humor. This is one to keep on the nightstand!"

—Pam Novotny, author of *The Joy of Twins and Other Multiple Births*

"This book was so exceedingly useful, I was implementing its tips just ten minutes after I cracked the spine. I'm glad I have *Twin Set,* though I wish it had been published two years ago to coincide with my twins' birth."

—A. J. Jacobs, author of *The Year of Living Biblically* (and father of twins)

"*Twin Set* is an engaging book chock-full of solid information, written by moms who have lived what they teach. The authors share countless tricks and tactics for surviving the challenges of multiples so that the whole family thrives. A must-read for dads as well as moms!"

—Dr. Linda Sonna, psychologist, professor, and author

TWIN SET

TWIN SET

MOMS *of* MULTIPLES

Share Survive & Thrive Secrets

CHRISTINA BOYLE
& CATHLEEN STAHL

THREE RIVERS PRESS • NEW YORK

The material in this book is for informational purposes only. As each individual situation is unique, you should use proper discretion, in consultation with your pediatrician, before utilizing the information contained in this book. The authors and publisher expressly disclaim responsibility for any adverse effects that may result from the use or application of the information contained in this book.

Library of Congress Cataloging-in-Publication Data

Boyle, Christina.
Twin set : moms of multiples share survive & thrive secrets / Christina Boyle and Cathleen Stahl.—1st ed.
p. cm.
Includes index.
1. Twins.   2. Child rearing.   3. Infants—Care.   4. Pregnancy.
I. Stahl, Cathleen.   II. Title.
HQ777.35.B68 2008
649'.144—dc22   2008000378

ISBN 978-0-307-39352-4

Printed in the United States of America

Design by Ruth Lee-Mui

10 9 8

First Edition

For T and R

—CB

For Jack and Emmet

—CS

CONTENTS

CONTENTS

INTRODUCTION

What lucky parents we are: we get twice the smiles and twice the I-love-yous. What a unique and wonderful gift we've been given: to observe and nurture the special bond that our twins have. And we are part of a phenomenon. According to the Centers for Disease Control and the National Center for Health Statistics, the twin birth rate is approximately 34 out of every 1,000 births in the United States. The national twin rate in the United States has risen 74 percent since 1980 and is expected to continue to rise at a rate of 2 percent annually for the next several years. We estimate that by 2010 there will be 1.3 million sets of young twins cruising around America.

Yet parenting young twins can feel like a truly singular experience.

Having had singleton children first (Christina has one older daughter and Cathy has two older sons), we've seen firsthand how raising our own twin sets is markedly different. The blessings— and the challenges—seem to grow exponentially, rather than merely doubling. Many of our tried-and-true parenting strategies just haven't translated to twins.

On the tough days, we've been hugely comforted by the support we've found in each other (we've been friends for years) and the other mothers of multiples in our community. Hearing advice from someone who's in the twin trenches and really "gets it" has been crucial to our evolution as moms of twins. Our hope is that this book assures you that you are not alone, and that this will be a place where you can find ideas, advice, support, and laughs.

To cast the widest possible net for the best twin parenting tips, we conducted a survey of more than three hundred moms of multiples from around the country. The moms who responded represent a variety of personal circumstances: some work, some have other kids, some have triplets, and some have multiple sets of multiples. Regardless of their background or location, these moms of multiples were all eager to share the kind of advice moms generally pass on to each other at the community playground or while waiting in line at the grocery store. This unique, connective, candid dialogue, which we call the mommy pipeline, is what we've tried to re-create on these pages. Whenever you need a point of reference from which to develop your own twin parenting strategies and techniques, we hope you'll consider this book a worthy girlfriend substitute.

We know from experience that even the most popular parenting philosophies won't work for every family. With the divergent and constantly evolving needs of twins, you need a stash of ideas to help you get through the day; what works one day may not work the next. When we've been out pushing our double strollers, many strangers have reacted to us with a mix of empathy and fascination. We've heard "I don't know how you do it" a lot—and so have our survey respondents. But as parents, we don't want to simply survive the challenge of parenting young twins. We want to thrive. The reality is that we probably end up somewhere in the middle, a parenting state we like to call "thrival." This is your thrival guide—the best ideas and tips vetted by hundreds of people who truly get it.

MEET OUR EXPERTS

MOMMY DOC

Dr. Lori Storch Smith, M.D., F.A.A.P., is a general pediatrician at Bay Street Pediatrics Associates, PC, in Westport, Connecticut. She served as president of Mothers of Multiples of Lower Fairfield County in Connecticut from August 2004—June 2007. She is the mother of girl/boy twins and a singleton girl and a singleton boy.

DADDY DOC

Dr. John E. Moore, M.D., F.A.A.P., is a general pediatrician practicing outpatient pediatrics for the Carillion Clinic in Roanoke, Virginia. He has written several articles on twins for pediatric journals, including *Contemporary Pediatrics* and *Pediatrics in Review*. He is the father of fraternal twin girls.

Roger B. Newman, M.D., is vice chairman of the obstetrics and gynecology department and director of the Twins Clinic at the Medical University of South Carolina.

Shirley M. Griffith, A.P.R.N., is a women's health nurse practitioner at Maternal Fetal Care PC in Stamford, Connecticut, where she has worked with partner (and husband) Dr. Richard Viscarello to deliver approximately three hundred sets of twins, seventy-two sets of triplets, and two sets of quads.

Soniyu Perl, M.S., R.D., is a nutritionist and mother of three, including fraternal twin girls, in Malibu, California.

Ciara Thurlow, a New York City–based personal stylist and founder of CPT Styling, is a mother of three, including fraternal twin boys.

John Gugle, CFP, CRPC, NAPFA–Registered Financial Advisor, principal, Alpha Financial Advisors, LLC, is a father of four, including fraternal twin boys, in Charlotte, North Carolina.

TWIN SET

Their Thrival

Depends on

Yours

1

PREGNANCY

finding out that you're having twins is the double surprise of a lifetime. Whether you've conceived them spontaneously or with some medical assistance, it's a big leap to go from longing to have one baby to knowing that you are going to be responsible for two. You are suddenly initiated into a very special club of mothers, one that seems to be expanding steadily. If you live in Connecticut, Massachusetts, New York, or New Jersey, you may feel like you see a lot of twins, and you'd be right. These states are known to have higher twin populations than the rest of the country. The twin trend is on the rise in Canada, the United Kingdom, and Australia as well.

Experts attribute the rise in twin birth rates to several things: moms are having babies later (after thirty-five), which means they ovulate differently and may produce two separate eggs during a cycle; moms are relying more on fertility medications (such as Clomid, which can increase your chance of having twins to one in ten); and moms are often using assisted-reproduction technology such as in vitro fertilization (IVF), which commonly transfers more than one embryo. (About 60 percent of the moms who took our survey used some sort of fertility treatment to get pregnant.)

But no matter how prepared—or unprepared—you were for the possibility of twins, you now have several months of lead time to take care of yourself properly, get the bare basics for their nursery, educate yourself on what's unique about having twins, and get excited about the babies you are going to have.

As both of us know from experience, a twin pregnancy is hands down way more demanding than a singleton pregnancy. Physically, you may be gaining more weight, carrying more baby weight, and experiencing the side effects of hormonal turmoil, such as heartburn (which can start as early as 20 weeks). Mentally, you may be riddled with practical worries ("Are their car seats going to fit in our car?") or forced to switch from a languid, easy-going mind-set to breaking down your life into weekly components. Emotionally, your moods may shift from bliss to panic, depending on how you feel physically or what twin thing you are thinking about. It can be even more nerve-racking if it's your first pregnancy. Luckily, the Twin Set Moms have some hard-won advice on how to keep your pregnancy feeling more blessed than stressed, even when the emotional stakes are high.

FIRST TIME, DOUBLE TIME

Being pregnant for the first time is an unbelievably special period in a woman's life. Everything is new, and there's a lot to learn and get excited about. If you are pregnant with multiples for your first pregnancy, it's a big deal and deserves to be cherished, celebrated, and respected. Blood tests, sonograms, and screenings can all bring you happy news, but they may also present an element of uncertainty as to the health of your developing babies. It's normal for any newly pregnant mom to freak out about a questionable or confusing test result, and probably even more so for a woman carrying multiples. Remember, you have a great reward waiting for you at the end of this marathon pregnancy, and that is two sweet babies who have nothing but love in their hearts for you. Still, it's important not to keep your worries bottled up inside; it's not good for you or your babies. Rather, share your concerns with your partner and your obstetrician. Sometimes, all any pregnant mom needs is a reassuring word to put your mind at ease and to help your body get the rest you require.

Are You Automatically Defined as "High Risk" When You Are Pregnant with Twins or More?

Dr. Roger Newman's opinion is yes. "Twins can have various complications that increase the risk of something going astray." According to Dr. Newman, virtually every potential obstetrical complication is magnified with multiple pregnancies. For instance, the average birth weight for twins is 5 pounds, as opposed to 7 pounds with singletons. Some general OB/GYNs prefer to follow their patients' twins themselves and watch them carefully for the development of such potential complications, referring them to a "high risk" specialist or perinatalogist for additional care. Cathy's OB managed the beginning of her twin pregnancy just as he did her singleton ones until she was about sixteen weeks. Then he had her visit a perinatalogist for monthly ultrasounds (sonograms). At the beginning of the third trimester, Cathy had sonograms every two weeks until thirty weeks, and then weekly ones until she delivered at thirty-seven weeks.

Nurse Shirley Griffith says that most perinatalogists work for hospitals and run a small department for consultation and ultrasounds. "Very few do deliveries," according to Griffith. "The most common reason that a patient is referred to a perinatalogist is for a level two ultrasound and possible chromosome testing, due to advanced maternal age (thirty-five and older)," she adds. If you would like more information on being seen by a high risk specialist, talk to your OB about it.

"Different" doesn't necessarily mean bad in the context of twin versus singleton pregnancy. Some differences are awesome, others not so much. For us, these were the biggies:

- **More doctor's visits and sonograms.** Addictive! Both of us were fortunate enough to have obstetricians who were exceptionally familiar with multiple pregnancies and births. Even though our doctors and nurses had seen their fair share of multiple mommas, our radiologists still oohed and aahed with us during our sonograms, and our nurses laughed as we groaned about getting on the scale. If you are a working woman, you may need to give your boss a heads-up that you'll probably have to duck out of the office a bit more frequently; if you are a stay-at-home mom, you may need to figure out what to do with your kids. You can plan for the frequency of both your doctor visits and sonograms to escalate as your pregnancy progresses. Dr. Newman breaks it down:

  First trimester. The first sonogram is usually when the radiologist figures out that there are two babies in there instead of one.

  Second trimester. Usually between eighteen and twenty weeks' gestation, you'll be given an ultrasound to check if the twins are developing properly. Dr. Newman adds, "At this scan we also check for the mother's cervical length measurement to try to assess her risk of preterm delivery. There is a significant direct relationship between cervix length and gestation length." Around twenty-four weeks, "we scan the patient again, and repeat the transvaginal cervical length measurement."

  Third trimester. "We will usually follow the twins' gestation on a monthly basis with ultrasounds in order to assess growth."

- **More glimpses of babies' personalities.** Awesome! The extra sonograms meant that we had the added bonus of seeing Baby A and Baby B interact. You may find that Baby A hogged more room in the beginning, yet Baby B kicked his or her way into position two weeks before delivery day. Some of the personality traits you notice in vitro may be consistent with what you see after your twins are born. For example, Christina's sonograms showed that Baby A was her son and Baby B was her daughter. Baby A was born first and almost a pound bigger. Baby B was often scrunched up on the sonogram and harder to see. Baby A is currently a loud and friendly child, and Baby B is a bit shyer and snuggly. Cathy's Twin A was dominant in utero, taking up the majority of space and literally pushing Twin B into a small corner. True to form, Twin A pushed out first and has been running the show ever since.

- **More pampering.** Awesome! Despite the growing twin birth rate, people tend to be in awe of a woman doing double time. You may get a pass on making side dishes for Thanksgiving and instead be brought second helpings by your grinning father-in-law. You may look more pregnant than you really are, but the visibility of your belly may mean that folks you don't really know are more courteous (holding doors for you and giving up seats on the bus). Trust us, you'll miss this after you give birth and you are out and about by yourself (probably doing a drugstore run) and the people treat you just like everyone else!

- **More pressure "down there."** Uncomfortable. In her seventh month of twin pregnancy, Christina felt as though her uterus was just going to drop out, especially at the end of a long day caring for her active preschooler. Despite all the pressure, the medical advice of her doctors was a laid-back "take it easy." When the pressure got too intense, she'd try to sit down for a few minutes and elevate her feet (she'd usually have to park her daughter in front of the television first). Other moms are more proactive about the intense pressure: they wear maternity belts, which come in a variety of styles and have an adjustable waist secured by Velcro and a back-support panel (look for them on amazon.com or fitmaternity.com). Sizing is often based on your pre-pregnancy hip or pants size, so you may want to upgrade a size or two to accommodate your twin belly.

- **Less comfortable sleeping positions.** Annoying. When your belly starts getting really big, typically around six and a half months (which is earlier than for singleton moms-to-be), you start fantasizing about sleeping on your belly (or on your back) again. To maximize her sleeping comfort, Cathy bought a body-size pillow (you can get them in The Company Store catalogue), slept on her left side, and wrapped her arms and legs around it (she was desperate for leg support at the end of a long day). These big, long pillows help stabilize you and keep you from teeter-tottering in bed.

- **More digestive issues.** Gross. The combination of more hormones whirling around in your body and more babies taking up room in your belly can mean you can't tolerate foods you'd normally eat with no problem. Christina experienced bad heartburn in her last trimester of her singleton pregnancy, but that was successfully combated with Tums and Pepto-Bismol. However, as early as her twentieth week of twin pregnancy, the heartburn showed up with a vengeance. By her third trimester, she was mixing prescription heartburn meds with over-the-counter products and eating her last meal of the day no later than three-thirty or four in the afternoon. Cereal and milk was about as spicy as she could take it.

- **More physically strenuous.** Exhausting. If only we'd known that we were going to be pregnant with twins, we would've gotten ourselves in much better shape first. Our doctors cut us off from moderate exercise by twenty weeks, whereas we exercised into our ninth month with our singletons. To deal with the physical strain, we asked for more help with our other kids. You do what you have to do to keep your strength up and get your rest.

Twincidentals: When Your Expanding Butt and Belly

Are a Hot Topic There's something about being pregnant with twins that turns you into the subject of public discussion, like it or not. You may be asked questions about how much weight you are gaining or hear comments like "Oh, wow, you're bigger than a barn!" Despite the fact that the twin birthrate is on the rise, people are still in awe of the size of the belly. Don't let these comments bring you down. Remember, it's good for you and the two babies you are growing when you pack on pounds. The attention can be fun if you have the right attitude. And after your twins arrive, conversations will be more focused on their appearance than yours. In fact, we bet you'll be hearing lots of "Wow, you just had twins? You look great!"

TACKLING YOUR BIGGEST PREGNANCY WORRIES

There *is* potentially more to worry about with a twin pregnancy than with a singleton pregnancy. For one thing, it's more of a strain on a mom's body, especially on her cervix, and there are increased chances of early delivery. Experts say that about 50 percent of twins are born before thirty-seven weeks (which is considered full term, versus forty weeks for singletons). Our survey results were consistent: almost half of the moms said that their twins were born before thirty-seven weeks. Our purpose in sharing these statistics is not to scare you, but rather to let you know that no matter what you do right, the outcome may be out of your hands.

Although there are no preparatory exercises you can do to strengthen your cervix, you can take your pregnancy week by week. Crossing one week at a time off your calendar is a good way to get accustomed to compartmentalizing so the thought of having twins doesn't seem so overwhelming and so you don't find your-self worrying too far into the future about things beyond your control. The women in our survey shared some of the things they worried about most. If any of these things are keeping you up at night, check out our coping strategies:

Worry: How am I going to recover from a C-section while caring for two babies?
Solution: Just because you are having twins doesn't mean you are having a C-section. This is something you need to talk about with your doctor throughout your pregnancy. According to Dr. New-man, a vaginal birth is possible for mothers of twins when both twins are positioned head down, which is about 40 percent of the time, or when one twin is head down and the other is breech or transverse, which is about another 40 percent of the time. And miracles do happen. Christina, whose first child was delivered vaginally, was told during her third trimester of twin pregnancy that she might have to have a C-section. Around her thirty-sixth week, one twin was upside down and the other was sideways. By her thirty-eighth week they'd moved: both twins were head down and ready for a vaginal delivery. But this isn't always the case, and obviously, if you've had C-sections before, your chances of having one for the birth of your twins is very high. If it looks like you are going to have a C-section, you have to plan ahead and get some help for a few weeks so you can recover.

Worry: How am I going to deal with sleep deprivation when they're here?
Solution: It's brutal, but moms of multiples have all gone through it. You can survive alone, but having help is always better. As one of the moms in our survey shared, "I wish I knew enough to get help lined up ahead of time." That is one thing you can do. You should also read our "Sleep Strategies" chapter, page 93, to see what it takes to get twins on a predictable sleeping schedule and

our "Good Help" chapter, page 169, for tips on finding the right help for your budget and needs.

Worry: How am I going to feed two babies at once?
Solution: Read our "Chow Time" chapter on page 71 for tips on breast- and bottle-feeding. You can also look into breast-feeding classes before and after you have the twins. You may even want to line up a lactation consultant to visit you at home after your babies are born.

Worry: How am I going to get the rest I need during pregnancy if I am up at night worrying about everything?
Solution: Keep a stash of boring reading next to your bed (golf supply catalogues, second-language books, and tax laws should do it). Or keep a pad and pen nearby to jot down your fears or items for your to-do list. Sometimes, writing stuff down frees your brain and allows you to start to relax again. If you still can't sleep, talk to your OB about homeopathic or medical remedies.

EATING RIGHT—FOR THREE

Eating as well as you possibly can is something you can control and a direct way to take care of yourself and your incubating babies during your twin pregnancy. It's true, good nutrition correlates to higher birth weights and good intrauterine growth. But pregnancy is a nutritionally challenging period for your body in any case, and even more so when it needs to provide good nutrition to more than one fetus, so we've asked nutritionist Soniyu Perl to share her expertise.

Eat a balanced diet. Aim for a mix of whole grains, fruits and veggies, fats and oils, and quality protein foods that contain all the essential amino acids (meat, fish, poultry, eggs, and dairy products). If you can't stomach meat at your meals, combine beans or lentils with grains instead. Aim for at least six servings of full-fat dairy (8 ounces of milk or a 1-ounce slice of cheese) and four servings from the protein group. If you are on the go, pack snacks in the morning (such as nuts, dried fruit, cereal, and granola bars) and carry them in your bag.

Eat enough calories. There are recommended dietary allowances (RDAs) for pregnant women with singletons; however, no guidelines have been set for women carrying multiples. Perl says an average non-pregnant woman needs 1,800 calories a day, and a good goal for a woman pregnant with twins is 3,000 calories a day. That means three meals and three snacks a day. If you are underweight, you first need to gain enough weight to take you to the normal range for your height, then put on the amount recommended for your twin pregnancy. The normal-weight mom should aim for 40 to 56 pounds. If you are overweight, go for 38 to 47 pounds.

Drink enough water. According to Perl, water consumption is especially important when expecting multiples because dehydration can trigger contractions. Aim for at least eight 16-ounce glasses of water every day. Develop a system to make sure you get what you need: lay out the bottles of water you need to drink at the beginning of the day, or drink a tall glass at the beginning of every hour. Try flavoring the water with lemon, cucumber, or a dash of fruit juice if it gets boring or if you are having a hard time keeping it down.

Fight morning sickness. When pregnant with twins or higher multiples, you're more likely to have morning (or in some cases all-day) sickness than a woman pregnant with a singleton. This may be from the higher levels of hCG, estrogen, or other hormones in your system. If you are vomiting, you may need to use sports drinks such as Powerade or Gatorade to replace lost electrolytes. To minimize nausea, eat saltines or toast before you get out of bed. During the day, try ginger, an alternative remedy thought to settle the stomach and help quell queasiness. See if you can find ginger ale made with real ginger (most big-brand ginger ales aren't), or grate fresh ginger into hot water to make ginger tea. Some women find temporary relief with Preggie Pops and Preggie Pop Drops (available at threelollies.com). Vitamin B_6 has long been thought to ease morning sickness, which is the premise behind B-natal Green Apple Lozenges or B-natal Cherry-Flavored TheraPops (both available at ladytobaby.com).

Do Your Homework, Even if It's Scary

The moms who answered our survey tended to either rely heavily on twin pregnancy books and Web sites or avoided them at all costs because they were "too scary." Because you are reading this book, we assume you'd like to have some answers on hand in case you need them. Here's a list of the multiples-specific resources our moms found the most helpful.

Books

When You're Expecting Twins, Triplets or Quads: Proven Guidelines for a Healthy Multiple Pregnancy, revised edition, by Dr. Barbara Luke and Tamara Eberline (HarperCollins, 2004), was the book mentioned most often by our survey respondents, who appreciated the specific dietary guidelines. Dr. Newman and Nurse Griffith both recommend this book, too.

Ready or Not Here We Come, second edition, by Elizabeth Lyons (Finn-Phyllis Press, 2007), is a humor-infused read for pregnant moms by a mom of twins, which our moms enjoyed when they needed a laugh.

Having Twins: A Parent's Guide to Multiple Pregnancy, Birth and Early Childhood, revised third edition, by Elizabeth Noble (Houghton Mifflin, 2003), was popular as well. Our moms said they benefited from this author's emphasis on prenatal care.

Web Sites and Blogs

Try twinsetmoms.com (our candid blog); tripletconnection.org (the best site for moms of triplets, which offers membership, newsletters, online forums, plus pregnancy and new-parent packets); sidelines.org (great for moms on bed rest, especially if you want to be paired up with an online or phone buddy); and IVFconnections.com (has a thriving online bulletin board community of more than twenty-five thousand members).

Groups

The National Organization of Mothers of Twins Clubs (NOMOTC) is a non-profit organization founded in 1960 to promote the special aspects of multiple-birth children and child development. It has more than 420 member clubs (known to us as Mothers of Multiples clubs) and twenty-five thousand members in the United States You can join as soon as you find out you are pregnant. Here's what some clubs do: hold monthly meetings with experts who speak about twin issues, publish for-hire lists (online or in their newsletters, so you can scope out babysitters, housecleaners, and more), and coordinate play groups and bed rest outreach. See nomotc.org for more information about a club near you and lots of other helpful information.

THE BED REST CLUB

Like almost half of our survey respondents, Cathy and Christina were told by their doctors to "take it easy." This mandate was sometimes laughable as we chased our other kids down grocery store aisles or searched under beds for their must-have sleepytime snugglers. Yet 25 percent of our moms said they were put on bed rest, 10 percent were regularly monitored at home or in the doctor's office, and 12 percent were hospitalized. Dr. Newman estimates from his practice that 20 to 30 percent of his patients with twins have some degree of bed rest. If you haven't lived through it, it is hard to imagine the kind of chaos that forced stillness can bring to your life. For our survey moms on bed rest, connecting with other moms who've been there was essential, whether on the phone or online. They recommend that you turn to your local Moms of Multiples group and sidelines.org, their favorite resources. More bed rest survival secrets from the moms we surveyed:

1. **Follow doctor's orders.** Take your medicine, drink your water, sit on the couch, don't have sex—do whatever it takes to keep your babies from being born too early. Trust that your doctor is being conservative with good reason and not to torture you with boredom. You will be so busy when the twins are born, you won't remember what it feels like to be pregnant and bored to tears.

2. **Take advantage of technology.** If you have been prescribed an at-home contraction monitor, use it accordingly. One mom who answered our survey was allowed to take short shopping trips if she used a motorized scooter or wheelchair. Many moms said their DVR and computers provided hours of entertainment.

3. **Rally the troops.** Now's the time to start delegating. Our moms' strategies: make Grandma your chauffeur and have her drive you to doctor's appointments, put your husband on kitchen duty, let the members of your church cook for you every night for a month, and hire a cleaning company. One smart mom had her own dad (also her colleague) bring her work home from the office—along with a weight-gain shake.

4. **Get some busywork done.** Rather than sit idly, our moms say they made and addressed birth announcements, did lots of word-find puzzles, bought baby products by phone, did all of their Christmas shopping online, caught up on ten years' worth of photos and quiet projects, and rekindled a love for needlework and knitting.

Terrific Twinsights: Be moved by the poignant things these moms of multiples told us about keeping a positive attitude during bed rest.

- **Change your thinking from "me" to "we."** "I was on hospital bed rest for ten weeks. I was all about the babies. I am a very active person, but it was not about me. Pregnant moms need to understand that."

- **Keep it in perspective.** "I worked full time from my couch for five weeks. That was easier than having two babies in the NICU."

- **Pretend it's a job assignment.** "I attacked it like a project, thinking that if I could do the best possible job at being on strict bed rest, monitoring, taking all my meds, drinking all my water, and eating healthy, I would be able to give birth to two healthy, full-term babies."

- **Relish the quiet time.** "I sat outside and read when it was nice out. I'd cut tags off baby clothes and float in our pool on a raft. I knew the relaxation was the last for a long, long time."

- **Give yourself something happy to think about.** "I scheduled my weekly ultrasounds for Wednesdays so I had something to look forward to midweek."

- **Call for help if you're slipping off the radar screen.** "I had some days I thought I'd go crazy and cried a lot. I stayed busy talking on the phone, watching movies, and having friends come by."

- **Prepare to nest.** "I came downstairs once in the morning and stayed down there, close to a computer, couch, bathroom, and kitchen, until bedtime."

- **Think about how sweet new babies are.** "I took a walk one day down the hall to the nursery, even though I wasn't supposed to be out of my hospital bed."

Life goes on around you when you are pregnant with multiples, and it's hard, or in some cases almost impossible, to let it all go and just focus on growing your babies in your belly. That said, here are some ways the moms who responded to our survey stayed connected to the important people.

Dealing with Your Husband

Problem: *The doctor says no sexual activity at all (plus six to eight weeks of waiting after you have the twins).*
Solution: Acknowledge that it's a long time for you to wait, too. Hold hands on the couch, rub his back, and find other ways to be intimate and remind him that you are worth the wait.

Problem: *He's taking your pregnancy too casually.*
Solution: Take him on your next few doctor's visits and have your doctor chat with him.

Problem: *He's taking your pregnancy too seriously.*
Solution: You can keep him busy with assembling two cribs, two mobiles, and two dressers for the nursery. Find him a friend with twins—chatting with a dad who has been through twin pregnancy and birth could help assuage your sweetie's fears. (And check out our "Dad Support" chapter on page 57).

Dealing with Your Other Children

Problem: *Your other kids are acting up because you can't give them the physical attention they are accustomed to.*

Solution: Even a two-year-old can understand that Mommy needs to rest on the couch or else she might get really sick. Don't blame your physical limitations on the twins; just blame it on your health. It may also help to do little things that help them feel special, such as sending them sweet notes in their lunch box, snuggling with them at bedtime, and letting them wear what they want for a week. Don't forget to call in the grandparents to dote on them when you can't.

Dealing with Your Friends and Family

Problem: They don't offer to help; you have to ask first.
Solution: Keep on asking. Be specific about what you need and why you can't do things for yourself right now. Be sure to thank people profusely, even if they didn't do exactly what you wanted them to do.

Problem: You feel left out.
Solution: E-mail your pals or call your sister and schedule some low-key bonding time. If you sense that they are tired of hearing your twin-baby talk, focus on all of the exciting, wonderful things you are still interested in outside of babies, and ask them about their lives.

Dealing with Your Co-workers

Problem: You have to cut back on hours and office time.
Solution: Get familiar with the Family and Medical Leave Act and what other women in your company have done in similar situations that may have set a desirable precedent. Voice your willingness to work from home, pending your doctor's approval.

Extra-Special Twin Pregnancy Circumstances

Adoption

Three percent of the moms who answered our survey said they adopted twins. Some suggested reading anything by Lois Ruskai Melina as well as *Adopting After Infertility* by Patricia Irwin Johnston. We interviewed three moms who've adopted twins, and compiled their most helpful advice:

- **Be patient about the adoption plan.** If you've arranged with a pregnant woman to adopt right after the birth, be aware that carrying twins may mean that the normal range of emotions that a biological mom may experience—anything from guilt to relief, hope, or fear—are exacerbated.
- **Do as much as you can.** Once you have a contract with a biological mother, you can get involved with her health care. In some cases, you will get updates and medical records from the adoption agency. In other cases, you can pick up the phone yourself and chat with the biological mom. One adoptive mom says she called the biological mom three to four times a week. She was also able to accompany the biological mom to ultrasounds and stress tests and receive copies of medical records in person.
- **Be proactive after an international adoption.** One mom told us that when her twins came home from Russia, she and her husband had very little medical information about them. "What we did have was sketchy, and didn't seem plausible or even realistic. We requested copies of all medical records on the boys from the orphanage and hospital they stayed in for quite a lengthy period of time. Many of them made no sense, were probably written about children other than our boys, and were generally disjointed." To combat the lack of information, this mom took her twins to a pediatrician who specialized in international adoptions. "During their first week home, we spent an entire afternoon with our pediatrician. Both boys received immunizations, a complete physical, hearing and eye tests, blood tests, and developmental testing. We had additional physicals completed every month for the first year, along with recommended occupational therapy, physical therapy, and speech and sensory training. Over the last three years, we've seen a variety of specialists, many of whom we've insisted on seeing the minute anything seemed slightly amiss. We've often been overly cautious, but feel justified in doing so." To take their sons' health care even further, this mom says that they've recently hired an investigator in Russia to conduct a birth mother search. "We hope that she will be able—and willing—to talk about her own medical history and perhaps even the medical history of the birth father."

Surrogacy

Two percent of the women we surveyed said they had their twins thanks to surrogacy. We interviewed one mom who told us about her experiences with gestational surrogacy. Through an IVF, the gestational carrier was impregnated with this mom's eggs and her husband's sperm. Very often the carrier is someone the mom knows, but it is becoming more common to go through an agency that does medical screening and provides a legally binding contract. (There's another type of surrogacy, called traditional surrogacy, which typically involves the surrogate supplying the eggs and being artificially inseminated with the sperm of the father-to-be. This may be more emotionally complicated because the surrogate has a genetic tie to the babies.) Here are one mom's tips for getting involved with the gestational carrier's pregnancy:

- **Choose an OB that you like.** You want one who will communicate your worries and keep the surrogate on a healthy track. You also want to make sure the doctor knows you plan on going to the doctor's appointments with the surrogate and being at the delivery.
- **Be a cheerleader.** It's tough to be pregnant with multiples, so do what you can to boost the surrogate's spirits. That could mean calling every day or sending her interesting articles in the mail—whatever provides her with emotional comfort.
- **Keep her previous habits in mind.** If you can, discuss the surrogate's diet and activity levels before the IVF. If she eats things that bother you, such as hot dogs or undercooked meat, privately discuss it with the OB first, to see what he or she says. If there is a problem, let the doctor communicate the concern instead of you.

2

. . . .

PREEMIE CARE

. . . .

Y ou'll probably learn during your pregnancy that premature babies (born before thirty-five weeks) are a fairly strong possibility for all mothers of multiples. But most of our doctors give us a goal of carrying our babies to thirty-seven weeks, considered full term for twins (versus forty weeks for singletons). Part of the miracle of modern medicine, with its advanced screening capabilities and prenatal care, is that it enables many women to carry two babies in utero much longer than in past generations. But despite these advances and your most heartfelt effort, delivering twins early is a very real issue and a frequent event.

According to national statistics, twins are born at thirty-four weeks on average (remember that twins born before thirty-five weeks are considered premature). Furthermore, about 50 percent of twins spend some time in the neonatal intensive care unit (NICU), a special-care nursery for preemies and newborn infants with severe medical complications, staffed by doctors and nurses with specialized training. Our survey participants reflect the national statistics: more than 50 percent of respondents said that one or both of their twins spent time in the NICU. While there, babies might sleep in incubators and be hooked up to breathing ventilators, feeding tubes, or apnea monitors, making you feel like you have lost all control. But the good news is that the survival rate of premature babies in general is up considerably over the last few decades, which experts attribute to better technology and increased awareness.

The implications of these statistics—it is a very real possibility that your twins will be born prematurely—can be a lot to worry about, especially if this is your first pregnancy, if you've had a history of difficult pregnancies, or if you know you have an incompetent cervix. Our survey moms were all too familiar with these fears. When we asked what they worried about most when pregnant with their twins, 38 percent said growing two healthy babies, 24 percent said not delivering the babies prematurely, and 10 percent said staying out of the NICU. We'd like to remind you that it doesn't happen to everyone, although the numbers do dictate a certain level of awareness among twin moms-to-be.

THE EMOTIONAL IMPACT OF PREMATURE DELIVERY

Lacking personal experience with premature babies, we conducted a focus group of moms of premature twins (many of whom now volunteer for The Tiny Miracles Foundation [ttmf.org], a nonprofit group in Connecticut devoted to supporting parents of premature infants) to gain deeper insight into the strain and anxiety they face—and the hope that propels them forward. The emotional toll of the experience was a common theme. As one of the moms said, "I felt like a failure when my twins were born at thirty-five weeks and whisked away to the NICU." The truth is, you may follow your doctor's instructions to the letter, but that doesn't mean your body will cooperate. We can't reiterate enough: having your babies prematurely does not make you a failure.

In a recent survey of moms of premature babies conducted by *Babytalk* magazine and the March of Dimes (a national nonprofit organization dedicated to preventing birth defects, premature birth, and infant mortality), 64 percent of their respondents said they sometimes felt guilty for delivering early. In addition to feeling guilty, moms of premature babies reported feeling caught off guard or cheated and finding themselves in an emotional whirlwind. According to this survey, 46 percent said that they didn't really feel like a parent until they brought their babies home. Some babies spend months in the NICU, where nurses are the primary caregivers, and this exacerbates moms' feelings of helplessness. We've heard moms of premature twins use words such as *fear, anger, shock,* and *depression* to describe the variety of ways they felt when their babies were in the NICU.

Of course, not all premature twins have medical problems. It really depends on how early they are born and how successfully their medical needs are met. This book is not intended to replace the wealth of medical information a mom of twins can access, particularly when it comes to preemie care (check out marchofdimes.com for resources). However, when it comes to caring for your premature twins in and out of the NICU, we can offer you the unique Twin Set Mom brand of tried-and-true strategies, based on the twin-specific wisdom of our survey and focus group mothers. These moms told us how helpful it was for them to talk to other parents of preemie twins, because they were the most understanding of their unique circumstances and challenges, even more than their most trusted family and friends. They said it is definitely one of those experiences in life that you really can't understand unless you've been through it. We are hoping that their practical tips and insights will present you with comfort and an understanding of that important parent-to-parent connection.

One of the moms in our focus group said, "There is no preparation. You are thrown into this." Yet, upon further discussion, she did concede that there are some things you can do when you are pregnant with twins to prepare for the possibility of having premature babies. Here's the best and most practical advice culled from preemie experts.

Research your hospital. Talk to your OB about the likelihood that you'll deliver your twins early, and then find out which hospitals near you are equipped to deal with premature babies with serious medical needs. Not all hospitals are created equal when it comes to preemie care: they are rated from Level I to Level III, based on the type of equipment they have and the intensity of training their medical staffs have received. According to Dr. Newman, "In general, Level I hospitals are not prepared to care for babies of less than thirty-seven weeks' gestation. So if your nearest hospital is a Level I facility, you should not go to that obstetric practice if you are carrying twins. There are some Level II facilities with neonatal specialists and they tend to be able to take care of infants delivered at thirty-two or thirty-four weeks. But your best bet is to receive care from providers who deliver at a Level III facility, which includes an NICU capable of and experienced in caring for very low-birth-weight infants and other complications."

Line up some help. If you have the financial resources and the space in your home, you may want to consider hiring a baby nurse to help you care for your twins. A baby nurse is a trained child care provider who comes into your home to assist with the daily care of your babies when they first come home from the hospital. Baby nurses generally work twenty-four-hour days, so they are on call to help you at all times. A baby nurse can help you establish a routine for your babies, or continue the one they were on in the hospital, and provide breast-feeding support. If your twins are premature, it's very important that the baby nurse you hire has experience caring for premature babies. One of the moms in our focus group said that you should hire a baby nurse to start around the time that your twins would be full term (thirty-seven weeks), because this is most likely when one or both twins will come home from the NICU.

In our part of Connecticut, which has one of the highest twin birth rates in the country, moms have been known to hire baby nurses as soon as they find out they are having more than one baby. One mom, who ultimately delivered her twins prematurely, said she found and hired her baby nurse when she was twelve weeks pregnant. Originally, the hire was made to take some stress out of caring for twins and a preschooler, but it turned out to be more of a lifesaver than a luxury in the end. Her nurse started when her twins were four weeks old—one twin had just come home from the NICU, but the other was still in the NICU (for about four more weeks). The original plan was for the nurse to stay for six weeks (at $1,800 a week), but our friend convinced her to stay until the twins were six months (at a reduced rate once they started sleeping through the night). "We had money set aside for the first six weeks, and then we used money that we probably should not have touched. But we have no regrets. It was the best money we ever spent." (For more info about finding a baby nurse or other, less expensive forms of child care, see our "Good Help" chapter, page 169.)

If you have other kids to care for, line up child care plans that can be sprung into action on a moment's notice. Set up car pools, put the grandparents and neighbors on standby, and clear some space in the freezer for lasagnas that may be donated to your cause. This was important for all of the moms in our focus group, who all had other children to care for in addition to their babies in the NICU (one had seven others, including another set of twins).

Take a tour of the NICU. This may enhance your comfort level and confidence in your hospital and doctors, but prepare yourself: some of the babies are very small and some of the equipment looks intimidating.

Buy some preemie clothes. The moms in our focus group tell us that preemie clothes are hard to come by. If you have premature babies by surprise, you may not have a baby shower to provide you with essentials. You can buy preemie outfits online from gap.com, ittybittybundles.com, preemiesrus.com, preemie.com, and snuggletown.com. One of our focus group moms really broke the clothing needs down for us: If you have micro-preemies (born before twenty-six weeks and under 2 pounds), they can only wear NICU T-shirts (check out the marketplace pages of *Preemie* magazine to find online sources for these, including jacquispreemie pride.com and preemietees.com) and diapers that allow the medical staff to easily access their bodies and see their skin tone at all times. If you have preemies born after thirty weeks and heavier than 2 pounds, it is best to buy one week's worth of "weight-sized" preemie clothes online (try preemie-yums.com). These babies will need about three cotton hats, two or three NICU T-shirts, and two or three NICU bag sleepers for easy access and changing. Some hospitals will allow socks at this age and weight. When your preemies are approaching their last week or two in the NICU, you can begin to buy a week's worth of preemie clothes for after you bring your babies home, which includes three preemie bag sleepers, five preemie onesies, three preemie footies, two preemie hats, and four or five pairs of preemie socks. These clothes will be too big on them for a while, and will probably last for the first six weeks at home. As a final tip, our mom says, "Put

Twincidentals: When Two Preemie Babies Need Care in Two Different Places

According to the moms in our focus group, within twenty-four hours of your twins' birth, you may find out that one or both are going to the NICU. This presents a logistical problem if one twin is released home before the other. Many of the moms from our survey encountered this dilemma. The length of their twins' stay in the NICU varied considerably, depending on their babies' medical stability. What's more, a couple of moms from our survey said that one or both of their babies spent time in different hospitals, depending on what kind of care they required and what the hospital was capable of dealing with. One incredible mom from our survey revealed that she had to travel 120 miles each trip for three weeks when one twin was sent to a different hospital that was better suited for that baby's medical needs.

If you find your preemie twins coming home at different times, or in different hospitals, you can't be on duty for both twins round the clock, because you will crash and burn. Not to mention you have a pregnancy and delivery to recover from. Split up the hours with Dad, so that one of you is able to be in the NICU as much as reality (your other kids, your jobs, your financial situation) allows, and one of you can get some rest or spend time with your other children at home. Many NICUs will also allow grandparents to visit the babies, so fit them into the schedule if possible.

a laundry bag on the side of your babies' incubators and label all their clothes." Something as simple as supplying your tiny babies with clothing and washing the clothes at home may give you some sense of reassurance and control.

The moms in our focus group emphasized that the NICU nurses are your greatest allies when it comes to figuring out how to care for your premature babies while they are in the hospital. Even if the nurses are busy, it is up to you to ask questions or share any concerns. Here are several other strategies.

Get familiar with your babies' limitations and restrictions. These will be dictated by their gestational age and their medical stability. Each of your babies may have a different set of problems, even though they are the same gestational age.

Know when you can be involved. In most cases, if your babies are thirty-four or thirty-five weeks and medically stable, you may be able to feed, hold, and bathe them. If you have micro-preemie babies, you may not be able to feed or touch them, especially if they are on a ventilator or need oxygen assistance.

Take charge of the feeding schedule. If your twins are in the same NICU, talk to the nurses about helping you manage their feeding schedule. It might be helpful if they are staggered by a half hour so that you can help feed and change each baby, assuming they are medically stable enough for that contact with you.

Set yourself up for breast-feeding success. Your breast milk is one of the greatest gifts you can give your babies. Since so much of your preemie twins' care may be out of your control, getting your breast milk supply up and running may be something you want to take charge of. According to a recent poll conducted online by *Preemie* magazine, 35 percent of respondents said they breast-fed in the NICU and/or after discharge with the help of supplements/formula, 33 percent breast-fed in the NICU and at home, and 7 percent were unable to breast-feed in the NICU but breast-fed exclusively after discharge. The NICU nurses will help you get a hospital-grade pump that you can use when you visit your preemies (you can rent one to take home). Consider hiring a lactation consultant to follow up with you when you get home. Keep in mind that most preemie babies aren't born ready to nurse because their suck-swallow-breathe coordination isn't developed until their due date.

Start kangaroo care as soon as you can. This means holding the preemie baby naked, with just a diaper, directly on the parent's bare chest. Blankets are then placed over the baby for warmth. Parents should always wear button-front shirts in the NICU so they can perform kangaroo care. This helps you and Dad bond with your babies more, and it teaches your babies how you smell. The smell of your breast milk will also help your babies gain weight and lower their heart rates, and it is proven to increase their survival rate. Your skin can also transfer antibodies to your twins' skin.

Realize that they can twin-bond when you get them home. You may not be able to have your twins be in contact with each other in the NICU, even though studies show it can be physiologically beneficial to both of them. A double twin incubator is a huge hospital expense (cost is upward of $100,000), so they are rare. Besides, your twins may have different body temperature needs and may be better off in their own incubators.

Recognize the light at the end of the tunnel. Your twins will be able to come home when they can suck, swallow, and breathe without interruption, maintain a healthy body temperature outside the incubator, and gain weight on their own. Our focus group moms joked about the best thing about babies being in the NICU is that they had been so used to a schedule it was almost easy to implement it when they finally got home.

Daddy Doc: What Is Adjusted Age and How Long Is It a Factor?

Moms of preemie babies may find it helpful to take their child's prematurity into account with regard to development and weight. After all, Daddy Doc says, "it isn't fair to expect a premature baby to meet milestones at the same rate as a full-term infant. They did not get the benefits of a complete forty weeks' gestation before they were born, and as such will not be meeting milestones at the same rates. For example, a two-month-old full-term baby will begin smiling, laughing, and holding her head up, while a two-month-old thirty-two-weeker will just be at her predicted at-birth levels of behavior." To adjust your preemies' age, go backward from their chronological age to their gestational age. A six-month-old baby who was born at thirty weeks has a corrected age of four months. Ideally, your preemies will narrow the gap between their two ages as the months progress and finally get caught up by the time they are two years old, unless they have delays for other reasons. When we asked our moms of preemie twins at what point they will feel that their preemie twins will have caught up with other kids their age, 39 percent said soon after they came home from the hospital; 29 percent said by one year; and 28 percent said two years.

Take it from the moms in our focus group, you are going to have to find ways to look after yourself and get physically strong again. Here's how to get started.

Ask for help. You may experience post-traumatic stress, but it may not happen until your twins have been home for a few months. Signs to look out for are being unable to sleep (even when your twins are), dramatic weight loss, and the inability to stay focused on priorities. If this sounds familiar, you have to see a doctor and get better. You can't take care of your twins if you are a mess.

Share your money woes. If you can't afford to pay for gas to travel to an NICU that's a hundred miles away from home, tell your hospital social worker. If you can't afford to pay for a baby nurse or babysitting when your twins first get home, assign a friend to research local senior centers for qualified programs where grandparents are caregivers. The point is, cast a wide net and be creative—you and your preemie babies deserve the support.

Tackle things bit by bit. If you think about all the chaos that having preemie twins causes in your life, you may freak out. Therefore, we recommend turning off your phone when you are home, accepting all meals that your neighbors make, and having your husband or a close friend manage CarePages for you. CarePages is a free online service that helps you update family and friends on your babies' health (for more info check out carepages.com).

Seek support from those who have been through it. Get connected through your chapter of Mothers of Multiples, see what the March of Dimes' parent support can do for you, and check out *Preemie* magazine.

Be realistic about your relationship. Remember that this is the worst possible circumstance for both you and your partner. He is probably so scared that he will do something wrong, and you may be fighting with him because he doesn't know how to begin to help you. Our focus group moms advise that you don't go with him to the NICU; rather, have him go before or after work and let him learn from the nurses, not from you, how to care for the babies. He will create his own bond with them. Plus this will give you time to rest or hang with your other kids at home.

Be realistic about your friends and family. There's no way they can understand what you are going through. But they can help out physically by keeping your house running and pampering your other kids.

LIFE AFTER THE NICU

It will be a happy day indeed when both twins are finally home from the NICU and you can really begin taking charge of their care and nurturing their twin bond. One mom in our focus group said, "All I cared about when they got home was that the twins slept together in one crib." Even if they don't sleep well together because they are so used to sleeping apart, that doesn't mean they won't bond.

While you should enjoy finally seeing your twins interacting and out of the hospital, there are two main stressful things about caring for premature twins at home that you should be mindful of.

Germs. According to our survey, the number one challenge in caring for preemie twins is the very real threat that common germs pose to their health. To tackle the germ issue, you have to be completely proactive and militant during the first one or two winters (when viruses are more prevalent) about having everyone around the twins wash their hands. One of our moms had to teach her older daughter to take off her shoes, wash her hands, and change her clothes as soon as she got home from kindergarten because her twin sisters had very delicate immune systems. Other moms have to restrict their other kids from having play dates, unless it's nice out and the older kids can all stay outside while the twins are napping inside. Another said she had bottles of Purell hand sanitizer everywhere imaginable. Our focus group moms agreed that you can't expect your friends and family to understand your germophobia. In fact, one of them said she got flak for not parading her twins around during the Christmas holidays (the height of sick season). Family and friends might think your ordeal is over simply because the babies have been released from the hospital. But they're wrong. Remember, you're in charge of managing social expectations and putting your twins' health above all else. You may be able to ease up on germ patrol after your twins are one or two years old.

Managing complex schedules. Not only do you want to keep the twins in sync, you have to feed them on a fixed plan (probably prescribed by a doctor), and you have to make sure they get the medicine and doctor's visits they need. Depending on your twins' medical stability, you may be visiting your pediatrician at least once a week for the first two months. If you are breast-feeding, it may be recommended that you bring them in more often to make sure they are adequately gaining weight or that you buy a medical-grade scale that you can use daily at home. Depending on where you live and what your health coverage is like, you may even have doctors and nurses visit the twins at home for the first few weeks. According to our focus group, it's not uncommon for premature babies to see a series of specialists to address ongoing health problems. This means you may have to bring both twins to all these appointments, even if only one needs to go. It could be another good reason to have some backup babysitting help.

GETTING EXTRA HELP FOR PREEMIE TWINS

If you are concerned that one or both of your preemie twins will have developmental issues, you can look into the Birth to Three program that your state offers. Generally speaking, an expert will come to your home to evaluate your twins and suggest what kind of therapy, if any, could be beneficial (most likely physical, occupational, or speech-language therapy). If one or both of your twins qualifies for Birth to Three, the cost of the therapy may be based on a sliding scale that factors in your adjusted gross income. For more information, see birth23.org.

According to one of our focus group moms, the *Twins* magazine book called *Special Report: Premature Twins and Triplets* is the best source for parenting preemie twins. For more sources of information and help go to ttmf.org and the Twins' Mall at twins magazine.com.

Terrific Twinsight: "We are just so grateful they are alive that we are softer on them. My twins can be brats, but we give them more leeway," one mom confesses. She says she and her husband will toughen up when the twins are in elementary school.

3

MOM CARE

Our hope for you is that you enjoy, not just survive, your days with twins, but we know there will certainly be times when you wouldn't describe yourself as completely thriving. We urge you to aim for the more realistic goal of somewhere in between—the thrival zone. We consider this thrival concept the heart of twin motherhood and your secret weapon when it comes to mommy care. Some days in the thrival zone may mean you are in your pajamas until you shower at night and put on clean ones. But other days, you may be up before the twins, paying bills, returning e-mails, doing yoga, putting on makeup, and then heading out the door with them for a fun-filled play date at the park.

How each day with twins turns out can feel like a roll of the dice, but if you have some basic routines and systems in place, you can stack the odds in favor of your thrival. Remember, you're better able to care for your twins when you're taking good care of yourself.

Life with twins can make it hard to get in a healthy groove. Often we opt for the convenience of take-out, drive-through, or prepared foods, without really thinking about how healthy they are. And although it's hard to find the time to plan and prep healthy meals, that's exactly why it is essential for you to put eating right up at the top of your to-do list: eating well gives you the energy you so desperately need to keep up with your twins and the rest of your duties. And it will help provide adequate nutrition when you are nursing, keep you healthy and calm, and lose the baby weight when you're ready. We've found that when we are in a healthy eating pattern, we feel more capable and less overwhelmed, even when life is chaotic. So we'll take the extra time to chop fresh veggies and grill some organic chicken for a salad at lunch, instead of skipping it or eating half a can of Pringles. But we've had weeks or months as moms of twins where we've felt yucky, tired, and stressed and eaten handfuls of our twins' Goldfish for dinner or their leftover chicken nuggets off their high chair trays. It's not easy to pull yourself out of a poor-eating slump, but it's so worth it when you start to feel and look better.

With the help of nutritionist Soniyu Perl, we share sound bites of advice for eating right that any mom of multiples can follow.

Leave water, water everywhere. You need to stay adequately hydrated when you are producing milk for your babies. If you are producing 40 ounces of breast milk a day, you'd need at least 40 ounces of extra water just to make the milk. This doesn't take into account your body's own daily need for water. You'll lose a lot of fluid during those first few postpartum weeks, and you may be peeing like a racehorse. But that's not a signal to cut down on your water consumption.

Three Ways to Make It Easier to Drink H₂O

1. Write yourself reminder notes and leave them where you will see them.
2. Designate a regular nursing or pumping spot that is stocked with water and snacks.
3. Buy water bottles in bulk so you can grab them and go.

Fuel your body. Moms who are nursing twins need to make sure they are getting adequate calories to sustain their milk-making abilities. The Recommended Dietary Allowance established by the Food and Nutrition Board of the National Academy of Sciences for a mother nursing a singleton is an extra 500 calories per day, which would take her to a total of about 2,200 calories. There are no current national dietary guidelines for women breast-feeding multiples. A total of 3,000 calories is recommended by Perl for mothers exclusively nursing twins. To help you conceptualize what a day's worth of 3,000 calories looks like, Perl created the chart below:

	REGULAR DIET (1,800 CALORIES)	BREAST-FEEDING TWINS DIET (3,000 CALORIES)
Breakfast	1 bowl of cereal with nonfat milk, 1 piece fruit	2 scrambled eggs with 1–2 slices bread, 1 glass milk, sliced cheese on the toast, 1 piece fruit
Late morning snack	A handful of grapes or some crackers and water	Cheese sandwich or almond butter and jelly sandwich with a glass of milk/milk shake
Lunch	Large salad, chicken/tuna sandwich	Tuna sandwich on a whole-grain bagel with a slice of tomato and lettuce, cole slaw or potato salad, juice

	REGULAR DIET (1,800 CALORIES)	BREAST-FEEDING TWINS DIET (3,000 CALORIES)
Midafternoon snack	Carrots and celery with dip or a banana	Crackers with cottage cheese, trail mix with dried fruit and nuts
Dinner	Salad, grilled chicken or salmon or lean meat, whole-wheat pasta, veggies	Broiled steak or chicken, baked potato with sour cream, Caesar salad, dinner roll, glass of milk, sliced strawberries
After dinner	Piece of chocolate	Ice cream sundae

Curb your caffeine enthusiasm. More than one-third of our survey respondents confess that they drink more than three servings of caffeine each day. (We do, too!) But nursing moms of multiples, no matter how tired, really have to watch the caffeine intake because it can accumulate in your infants' bloodstream. According to Perl, one cup of coffee will only leave low traces of caffeine in your babies' system, but those second and

Thrival Tip: If you are in the phase when you are having lots of meals donated from neighbors, friends, or your church group and you're not so sure how healthy they are, make sure, just as in pregnancy, that the calories you eat come from good sources. To boost any donated meal nutritionally, you can supplement with your own fruits and veggies. Perl guesses that most meals that are brought to you will have the protein and grain components you need already.

third cups, or the additional sodas or teas, can really add up. If your babies seem restless or hard to settle down for sleep, you may want to cut down on caffeinated culprits (chocolate and some over-the-counter medications have it, too) for two to three weeks. Even after your babies are settling down to more normal sleep patterns, you may still want to stick with herbal tea and diet Sprite, at least for a while.

Caffeine is also naughty because it's a known diuretic. If you are nursing, that means you need to consume extra water if you drink strong coffee or tea or caffeinated sodas. "Caffeine also inhibits calcium and iron absorption, which may contribute to osteoporosis and anemia in women," Perl adds. She also recommends avoiding some drinks that are marketed as "energy boosters," which have high amounts of caffeine. They can give you a temporary boost, she says, but "caffeine is not a nutrient and should be limited in the diet."

Befriend energy-boosting foods. We all know that carbohydrates boost energy. It's the kind of carbs you eat that make a difference in sustaining regular energy levels throughout the course of a twin-packed day. Refined carbs such as white bread, white pasta, and sugary drinks may jump-start your energy, but you will experience a sharp drop in energy after the sugar from those sources is quickly processed. According to Perl, better choices are whole-grain toast with a protein such as almond butter, or whole-grain pasta with a sprinkle of parmesan cheese. Combining whole grains with small to moderate amounts of protein is the best way to keep your energy consistent all day long.

Plan for future meals. Leaving your home to buy the ingredients you need to make tasty salads for yourself may not be feasible when your twins are first born (your C-section recovery may keep you from driving, or you may be too busy or tired to deal). When they are toddlers, it can be tough to find a store with a grocery cart that can accommodate two children. That means you may have to get creative to make your shopping options work for you.

To make sure her home is always stocked with healthy foods for her and her family, Cathy has implemented a grocery shopping routine as part of her hectic week. To keep her needs straight, she creates multiple lists (one for the wholesale club, one for the farmers' market, one for the grocery store). She also considers what she can cook for dinner that is relatively healthy and that all six family members will eat, and what will work as leftovers. Once she's finalized her lists and menu, she hits the stores. She tries to hit the farmers' market once a week for in-season produce—it's outdoors, so no carts are needed. She brings her own stroller. She goes to the wholesale club about twice a month for basics that her boys blow through, including organic milk and eggs, orange juice, bread, pretzels, and cookies. Once a week, she'll supplement or get specialty items at the grocery store. True, the planning involved feels like prepping for a shuttle launch, and it seems crazy not to just pick everything up at one store, but her organic drive plus the desire to save money runs too deep.

In some locations, you can shop online using Fresh Direct or Peapod, a shortcut that seems made for moms of twins. There's a time commitment during your first visit to the site, when you shop virtually and make your base list, which is then tweaked and tailored to meet your weekly needs. It may be hard to let someone else pick out your apples and lettuce for you, but if you are consistently getting good-quality produce delivered to your front door, you might get used to it.

Be patient with your post-babies bod. Moms of twins tend to gain about 20 more pounds than moms carrying a single baby. This translates into more weight to lose to get back into your sassy jeans. Perl, like us, gained more weight with her twin pregnancy than with her singleton one, and expects that it's going to take longer to lose it. She says she's trying not to focus on weight loss while she's nursing her twins. Another sanity saver is to try not to compare yourself to women who've had singletons around the same time your twins were born. "Some nursing women enjoy rapid weight loss," Perl says. "But others find that they lose those last stubborn 5 or 7 pounds after they've weaned."

Remember, you got two babies out of one body, so ease up on yourself. Your body will lose weight at a pace that's right for you, and recover from your twin delivery in its own way, too. Moms of twins have different healing times with a C-section, ranging from four to twelve weeks. Some feel mild soreness (around the surgical scar) for up to six months postpartum.

Before you start exercising again, check with your OB. Ease back into it by popping your babies in the double Snap 'N Go and hitting the pavement for a walk. Perl says you can also focus on gradually building your ab muscles by doing crunches. "You can find workout DVDs to use at home when the twins are napping," she adds. Or find a conveniently located gym that has a well-staffed nursery.

Perl says that most busy moms of multiples find taking the time to diet and eat well is easier than carving out time for exercise to help with weight control. However, she points out, both are essential to keeping the weight off forever. According to Perl, "Technically, there's no magic number of calories we should all eat each day to lose weight. Most people can lose weight eating around 1,500 calories per day. If you can put in cardiovascular exercise three times per week (a good starting goal is thirty minutes), you can be a little more lenient with calorie intake."

Perl offers these tips for losing the twin baby weight:

1. Focus on whole grains, fruits and vegetables, lean chicken, and fish, limiting (if you have the will) foods with sugar and white flour.

2. Start the day with high-fiber, low-sugar cereal such as Fiber One (choose a cereal that has at least 5 grams of fiber per serving) and non-fat milk. Throw in blueberries or strawberries for an added punch.

3. Have an early lunch with a nice large salad (Perl varies the greens and adds radishes, carrots, cucumbers, mint, cilantro, dried fruits, nuts, garbanzo beans, kidney beans, or chicken cubes) and have at least four different low-calorie dressings to choose from. Sometimes Perl will make herself a cheese sandwich or tuna sandwich (with whole-grain bread and low-fat cheese slices or light canned tuna) and eat it with seasonal fruit.

4. Make an extra effort, when eating out, to order grilled entrees and ask for a salad on the side. Take home half of the entree if it's too large because portion sizes are crucial when it comes to weight loss.

5. Seek help if you need it. Consider working with a nutritionist (your OB may even have one in his or her office), write down everything you eat in a food journal, and note when you eat poorly to see what your emotional triggers are. A diet buddy, a trusted friend to whom you will hold yourself accountable, might tip the scales in your favor, too.

6. Take a multivitamin. Talk to your physician about your diet and lifestyle to determine what kind of vitamin you should take. He or she may prescribe a calcium or iron supplement if a deficiency is detected.

Certainly, there are effective at-home methods of exercise to consider that you can incorporate when your twins are still sleeping in the early morning or napping in the afternoon. Some moms even bust a sweat after nighttime tuck-ins. Christina used to exercise at home on an elliptical machine when her twins were babies. When they were tiny, she'd plop them on the floor in their baby buckets and they'd watch her for a half hour. When they started crawling and cruising, she put them close by in a play yard. When they started pushing the play yard around her room and trying to climb out (around fifteen months), all bets were off. Plan B was trying to work out early in the morning. But the squeaks from her machine woke up her older daughter. Plan C was working out during the twins' nap time while her older child was at preschool. But the twins stopped napping around eighteen months. Plan D was finding a part-time babysitter during the week and getting Dad to deal with the kids for a bit on the weekends. You get the point: keep trying to find ways to make time for yourself. If there is a will, there is a way to be bootylicious.

Twincidentals: Exercising as Your Twins Get Older

When twins are little babies, planning a walk or jog with them in tow means considering their feeding and napping schedules. It often makes sense to put them in the double stroller right after they've been fed and changed. Sometimes baby twins will nap in the stroller while Mom feels the burn. As baby twins morph into toddler twins, convincing them to get buckled into the stroller may become more challenging. We've gotten all geared up to run or power-walk only to turn home after a block or so because of the in-stroller fighting or screaming. Bribery is one option ("I have a bag of chocolate Teddy Grahams for each of you if you sit down"), and threats are another ("If you don't let me buckle you in, you are going to get a time-out"). Neither is an ideal parenting move, but getting your workout in and blowing off some steam may be more important for your family's overall health and well-being.

DRESSING AND LOOKING LIKE
A HOT NEW MOM (MOM OF MULTIPLES)

After you give birth, giving yourself the gift of a wardrobe makeover may be an integral part of your thrival. Stylist Ciara Thurlow shares her savviest look-hot strategies.

First, purge your closet. That means putting away the empire-waist maternity tops and tent dresses. Baggy clothes don't hide bulges—they make you look like you're still pregnant. Luckily, you can be a little more lenient with bottoms. Slowly wean off wearing maternity pants, she says, but maternity jeans are another story. Her favorites, because of the way they are cut for a mom's transitioning body, are made by Juicy and Seven for All Mankind. Thurlow also suggests that you keep your pre-pregnancy clothes out of sight. There is no need to torture yourself with visions of your skinny jeans every morning. After you have cleared some space in your closet, it's time for some retail therapy.

Don't underestimate the underwear. Start by loading up on strategic underpinnings to hold in or smooth out your belly and back fat and push up your breasts (whether or not you are nursing). Thurlow raves about the smoothing power of GapBody camisoles, which come in black, white, and nude. She also recommends going to Target to find more structured undergarments, such as a padded underwire bra top that connects to a stretchy camisole bottom (she found one made by Hanes). Other underpinnings to consider: a postpartum wrap belt to provide gentle support after a C-section or vaginal delivery (Medela makes them), an upper-body girdle with flexible boning (she found one by Hanes), a lower-body girdle (the one she found was like the top of a pair of super support stockings), and a whole-body tube dress made of nylon and spandex by La Serja. One note about underpinnings: consider getting them in a size larger than you normally would, to avoid the dreaded muffin-top look (when your hip, tummy, and back fat bulges out over your waistband).

Score your transition wardrobe on a tight budget. Oftentimes, new moms who are trying to lose weight are told not to buy any transition clothes. The thinking is that it will distract you from getting your body back in peak condition. Thurlow disagrees with that notion and instead believes it is important for a new mom to dress in cute clothes (even if they're in bigger sizes than you are used to wearing) and feel good along the way to recovering your physique.

That said, not every mom has room in the family budget for in between mommy clothes. To keep costs lower, Thurlow recommends asking your stylish girlfriends who are a size or two bigger than you if you can borrow some of their clothes. Girlfriends are often very generous about swapping maternity clothes, so why not do the same with transition clothes? Or you can ask your girlfriends to forgo a gift for the twins and instead give you a gift certificate to Old Navy or Target. We know of some moms who have returned unnecessary baby gifts to department stores that carry adult clothes and picked up a couple of new things for themselves instead.

Where to Shop for Your Post-Twins Basics

- Discount stores like Loehmann's, Marshalls, or TJ Maxx
- Stylish yet affordable shops such as Old Navy, Zara, H&M, and Target
- Reputable Web sites such as eBay for shoes if your feet have grown during pregnancy

Four Style Tips for Every New Mom of Twins

1. **Stick with a neutral template and add color, flair, and trendiness with accessories.** A monochromatic outfit will be slimming, especially in darker neutrals such as navy, charcoal, chocolate, or black. Good accessories such as hair scarves, bracelets, long necklaces, shoes, and bags will draw attention away from your problem areas.

2. **Open your fashion mind.** Jackets aren't just for the office—they look cute taking a walk with the double stroller, too. And hoodies aren't just for workouts. Some are chic enough to double as daywear (the pockets have a surprising distracting effect from a middle bulge).

3. **Primp when you can.** Taking the time to do your makeup and hair can make you feel better about yourself and motivate you to keep trying to get back in shape.

4. **Find new style icons.** If you have new curves to embrace because of nursing and pregnancy weight gain, look at how gorgeous celebrities (and moms of twins) such as Jennifer Lopez and Marcia Cross appear at big events— pre- and post-twins. Their confidence is their best accessory. Lots of new celeb moms highlight their voluptuousness in a tasteful and sophisticated way.

Choose pieces that accentuate your postpartum positives. If you like your legs and want to hide your belly, consider above-the knee A-line or bubble dresses in structured fabrics such as crisp linen and cotton, wool, and tweed, or short dresses with pockets to hide the belly. Also, think about layered tops (start with a tight camisole or bodysuit and add a long tank and then a shorter tee) with a miniskirt. The point is to keep the line long, to give the illusion that you are leaner in the middle. If you need to dress it up for work, add a formfitting jacket on top. Thurlow suggests Theory jackets and dressy formfitting layering pieces. You can find them for less at Loehmann's or buy them on sale.

If you like your bustline and want to minimize your lower abdomen and hips, consider formfitting slacks, jeans, or pants and a long, lean tank with a shorter cardigan or hoodie to cover the lower belly. You can dress this concept up with a pencil skirt, pumps, and a structured button-front blouse. Wrap dresses also flaunt the bust and play down the hips.

Shower yourself with love. It's the oldest of mom jokes: when do you have time to take a shower? But a shower can bring an emotional cleansing, too. We always feel better. Showering—and good grooming and hygiene in general—sends a message to the world that you care about yourself. This extra self-esteem boost can be particularly comforting while getting used to our post-twins bodies and lifestyles. You may find that waking up before the twins is the only way to get your shower in. Or you might do it at the end of the day, with your toddler twins in bath seats. Sometimes you'll squeeze it in at midday while they are snoozing, or happily watching a video, or with your toddler twins waiting for you on the bath mat, ready to hand you a towel.

CATCH SOME ZZZS

If you are still in the new-babies phase of twin parenting, you are probably pooped. Almost half of the moms who answered our survey said that sleep deprivation was the hardest hurdle to overcome during the first three months after their twins' birth. In fact, one mom told us, "A prisoner of war probably gets more sleep than I got those first three months."

It is really hard to get one baby on a good sleep routine, and to coordinate with another baby is a mammoth challenge. But it can be done (see our "Sleep Strategies" chapter, page 93, for tips). In most cases, it takes several weeks or months for your routine to pay off and predictable sleep patterns to emerge with long stretches at night. While you are waiting for that magic to happen, you can embrace the joy of the nap.

Our survey moms said they basically had a "take it when you can get it" philosophy about getting their sleep. For some moms of multiples, it is hard to get used to sleeping during the day rather than at night. It can also be difficult to quiet the thoughts of all you could be doing instead of napping. For other moms, it's easy to nap while the twins are napping. When you're physically and mentally drained, shutting down for a half hour, an hour, or even two can be a quick fix to help you get through the rest of the day (and possibly night). Christina struggled with learning how to nap and rarely did so when her older daughter was born, but she knew she needed to give herself a break after being up all night with the twins. She started by making sure that someone else was in the house to be responsible for the twins if they woke up, and then used earplugs to block out background noise. To calm her thoughts, she'd repeat a mantra until that became the focus of her concentration.

Daytime Sleep Supplies

Eye mask. Block out daytime light and sink into a lovely state of sleep.

Alarm clock. If you are worried that you will sleep for days when finally given the chance, set an alarm and sleep worry-free.

Earplugs. These can diminish the sound of crying twins, but use them only if another responsible adult is on twin duty.

Soothing sounds. This could mean a fan or a white-noise machine from the Sharper Image. There are tons of CDs out there with recordings of rainfalls, tropical breezes, classical music, and mellow jazz. We've even come across a Power Nap Kit CD (available at powernapkit.com).

How Baby Twins Change Your Sex Life

Thirty percent of the moms surveyed said one of the best things the twins' daddy did to help them was "not trying to jump my bones for a while." Our survey respondents also shared how their sex lives have changed since having twins: one-third said: "Sleep has become the new sex for both of us"; one-third said: "After being touched by the twins all day it's hard to muster up the desire for affection"; one-fifth said: "I don't feel sexy anymore"; and the rest pinned a sexual decline on having "no room in the bed because the twins are there."

SLEEP IS THE NEW SEX

Returning to a sex life is part of a mom's post-twins recovery. When you have sex, certain "feel-good" hormones are released in your body, which can lead to a temporary surge in romantic feelings for your partner. Sex is healthy for the marriage on multiple levels, and for some of us, getting the OB's green light to have sex again (usually around six to eight weeks postpartum) is a welcome message. For other moms, it takes several more weeks or even months to feel ready.

Because moms of twin infants are so tired and overwhelmed, even the idea of returning to sex can seem like a big joke. Christina's doctor gave her the go-ahead at six weeks and then said, "If you need to, you can tell your husband that I said you need to wait a total of twelve weeks, six weeks for each twin." It's no joke, though, that lots of factors can contribute to moms of multiples' lack of sex drive. And we'd be remiss to exclude being out of practice. (Keep in mind that many moms are on bed rest— meaning no sex—while pregnant with twins.) To add to the tension, dads of twins are often sex-starved, beginning the last several weeks or months before their twins are even born, because their wives are on bed rest or just too huge or uncomfortable to get very physical. And many dads have to wait several more weeks or months after their twins are born to have some sexual encounter with their wives because of the physical postpartum recovery and the exhaustion of caring for new twins.

Another factor that may keep you from wanting to have sex is worrying that you'll get pregnant again. This is especially true for moms who had a tough pregnancy and delivery or who already have other kids. Cathy was lucky to have experienced the joy and shock of spontaneous twins, so she felt like a fertility goddess had her in her sights. She was afraid a mere handshake with her husband might lead to more babies. If pregnancy paranoia is keeping you from getting busy, it may be time to talk to your OB about your birth control options (including having your husband get a vasectomy, which one of our moms says is the best thing that happened to their post-twins sex life).

MAKING TIME FOR MOMMY

Since our twins are not our first kids, and since we both work in various capacities while rearing children, we know well how it feels to be stressed. There were many days and weeks when writing this book put us over the edge. Like many moms of twins, we describe ourselves as not just "busy" but "crazy." Almost half of the moms who answered our survey said they have broken down crying in the middle of the day because they feel overwhelmed. One mom told us, "It is almost staggeringly hard to be a mom of multiples. Hating your responsibility at times doesn't mean you don't love your kids." Another mom adds, "The cooking, feeding, and cleaning! My husband and I joke that we feel like employees at a motel, taking turns at being short-order cook and maid." On a similar note, one mom says, "It really is hard and never-ending work."

We are all too familiar with those moments of feeling we are getting nothing done, dropping lots of balls, and not doing anything particularly well except getting frustrated.

Your Get-a-Grip Guide to Busting Twin Mommy Stress

- **Acknowledge that moms of twins have stressful lives.** Daddy Doc says one study shows that mothers of twins have significantly higher levels of stress than singleton mothers or mothers with close-in-age kids.
- **Realize that sometimes this stress gets in the way of the easy, breezy, baby-on-your-hip fantasy you envisioned before you had twins.** While pregnant with twins, you may have said to yourself, "I am going to nurse them for twelve months" or "I am going to make sure they know they are special individuals." But sometimes the reality of caring for two small babies interferes with our best intentions.
- **Accept that it's common for moms of twins to feel guilty.** One of our survey moms admits, "I wish I'd known how quickly the first two years go. It's hard to remember the individual milestones." Twin mom guilt is pervasive: almost half of our survey respondents agreed that they experience strong feelings of guilt because they fear they are not giving enough to each child. One brave soul from our survey shared what makes her feel guilty: "The feeling that both twins were being cheated. Only receiving 50 percent of me, versus getting all 100 percent of me if they were singletons."
- **Get a grip!** We all get bogged down with the sheer weight of our responsibilities, twins and otherwise, but we can't let that stop us from trying to be the best moms we can be. So long as you continue to be aware of what kind of mom you want to be, even if you aren't quite there yet, that's half the battle. You are probably doing a much better job than you realize, which may be hard for you to gauge because you aren't getting a quarterly job performance review from your family.
- **Allow yourself to let some things slide.** One survey mom laments that her biggest parenting mistake was "worrying about the silly things like cleaning the house and straightening up" instead of spending quality time with her twins or doing something nice for herself.
- **Remember the rewards of your hard work.** Another mom appreciates the payoff of the challenges: "I wish I had known how hard it would be. But also how amazing it is to watch these two very different people grow into little girls who love each other so much. They can always make each other laugh and are totally aware when the other needs them." Even if you can't always be there for each of your twins, take heart knowing that they always have each other.

In order to feel less overwhelmed and frustrated, we've learned to make to-do lists and to keep our planners updated and consult them often. Having everything in one place gives us peace of mind, helps us run more efficiently, and increases our chances of finding time for a quick workout or a funny e-mail exchange with a good friend. If you do find yourself with some downtime (your twins are napping, on a playdate, out with Dad, or at school), you don't have to use it to get something done. We can't emphasize this enough: simply resting or relaxing is doing something—it's called taking care of yourself.

If you start carving out time for yourself, you will have more patience, energy, and fun to give your twins. For more than 10 percent of the moms who answered our survey, not having any downtime was the single most stressful aspect of having twins. As one mom said, "My biggest mistake was not taking enough time

Mommy Tricks to Make More Time for Yourself During the Day

Many survey moms with school-age twins rely on large whiteboards that list kid activities and family responsibilities. If you aren't rushing forgotten show-and-tell items to school, you will have time for the gym or for a call to a friend. Our survey moms also revealed some time-saving tips that helped create a little extra mommy time:

- **Skip the morning scramble.** "I laid out everything the night before—clothes, diapers, socks—and filled the backpack for the next day. I laid my clothes out, too."
- **Wake and primp.** "Get up before them to shower and have coffee."
- **Appeal to your viewing pleasure.** "TiVo lots of shows so there's always something to watch when nursing."
- **Put kids to bed early.** "We make sure we have all five kids to bed by eight-fifteen so we have time to ourselves. I take an hour at night to straighten up the house and prepare for the next day."

for myself and finding help in our community. I have had days where I am really irritated all day and that isn't fair to the twins." Here are two ways to get a break on a regular basis.

Build it into your daily routine. One mom says her biggest twin parenting success was "taking a little time for myself during the day by watching a show that I like on TV other than *Barney.*" Start with a few minutes of reading a great book or listening to your favorite music in the middle of the day. Get a phone with a headset and chat with your college roommate while you are folding twin laundry or washing sippy cups at the sink.

Get help so you can fly the coop. After you get a taste of what a few minutes of calm or fun are like, you'll be hungry for more. You might be ready to indulge yourself with a trip out of the house that's twin-free. If you have reliable backup, you can shop, hit the gym, get a manicure, or have a fantastic white mocha with caramel. When we asked our survey respondents what's the best thing the twins' daddy did to help you, 80 percent said, "He took the twins on a regular basis so I could have some time to myself." (Maybe he deserves more than a new tie for Father's Day?)

How Working Moms of Twins Can De-Stress

For working moms of twins, the laws of math are what get you. True, our twins provide more than twice the joy, but they also require more than twice the effort in terms of care and management. Adding job responsibilities to the equation means less time, one of the most precious mom commodities, and more mental pressure. You can't be in two places at one time, and when you are home, you need to split your time and energy between two demanding clients, your twins. It becomes really hard to find time for things such as exercising and spending time with friends. Something has got to give—and for many working moms of twins, it's typically you.

If you work part or full time, like 44 percent of the moms we surveyed, you are adding another layer to the onion of your life as a family with young twins. Sometimes that last layer adds the spice you need; other times, it makes you cry!

- **Start by caring for your peace of mind.** Find the right child care situation for your twins. If you know they are happy and safe, you'll work better and save yourself some mental anguish. There are many different options available for child care; see our "Good Help" chapter, page 169, for the pros and cons of these as they relate to the care of twins.
- **Get an assistant for the other parts of your life.** In all likelihood, you'll need many assistants. Ask your babysitter to be in charge of the twins' toys and clothes. Shift some of your traditional household responsibilities to your partner. Outsource things such as dry cleaning or grocery shopping wherever possible. The freer you are to be with your twins when you get home from work, the better you'll feel about juggling.
- **Work in time to care for the rest of yourself, too.** If you don't want to be away from your twins to go to the gym on your days off, then walk them in the double stroller. Talk to friends at night after the twins are asleep. Utilize e-mail or text messaging. They are not a permanent solution, but at least you'll know what's going on in your friends' lives, and it's a great way to make a date to see each other.
- **Become an organizational junkie.** Sometimes writing things down makes you feel as if you have more control over the situation and helps a working mom stay connected to the daily ins and outs of her twins' lives. Write out the daily schedule; pick out their clothes; plan their lunch menu even though you're not feeding it to them.
- **Allow yourself to splurge . . . on yourself.** Take a vacation day on a random Tuesday so you can take your toddler twins to their regularly scheduled music class. Once in a while, get a manicure with a few extra minutes on the weekend or during your lunch hour instead of running a family errand. Now and then skip your responsible approach and indulge. The mental reward of skipping out on a minor responsibility is a major rush.
- **Save money.** The best thing about working is that they pay you to do it. Working is mentally satisfying and enables you to provide financial support for the twin expenses.
- **Tap into your energy reserves.** One of our working moms of twins says there is a physical drain to working outside of the home. She admits "feeling

too exhausted at times to come home and play with the twins." Sometimes something as simple as changing into more comfy clothes could motivate you to slip out of work mode and into play mode. We hope a little backyard catch or game of hide-and-seek will give you a second wind.

THE POSTPARTUM EMOTIONAL ROLLER COASTER

According to 5 percent of the moms who answered our survey, postpartum depression (PPD) was the hardest hurdle to overcome during the first three months after their twins were born. One survey mom revealed, "I will never, ever forgive myself for the anger and frustration I felt toward my twins, despite knowing from parents, experts, etc., that's it's completely normal to feel that way." According to Dr. Newman, the risk of PPD is higher in moms of multiples compared to moms of singletons. "I would suspect that it is more common due to greater stress, greater fatigue, greater demands on the mother's time, and relatively few resources to turn to. Another contributor would be the much higher rate of premature births and the early separation between a mother and her babies. I would also suspect that there is a hormonal factor, in that there is a greater fluctuation between the antepartum and postpartum states. Some have attributed postpartum depression to a condition that results in a thyroid hormone deficiency, which is also more common in multiple gestations." A PPD diagnosis can be made anytime within the first year after your twins' birth. The duration of PPD is highly variable, depending on how soon it is treated and what kind of treatment you are using.

Although it is common for new moms to have the baby blues, characterized by crying, trouble sleeping, difficulty making decisions, and doubting your ability to mother, PPD is considered far more serious and long-lasting (two weeks or more). If you have PPD, you might have trouble doing daily tasks, panic attacks, a change in appetite, worries about harming your child(ren), or thoughts about harming yourself. If you think you have PPD, consult with your doctor as soon as possible. PPD is often treated with light box therapy, psychotherapy, support groups, and/or antidepressants. Different medications affect breast-feeding babies differently, so talk to your doctor about which medication would be best. For more information about PPD, check out mededppd.org, postpartum.net, womensbehavioralhealth.org, and acog.org.

4

DAD SUPPORT

Clearly, this book is written with moms in mind. But having twins is a big adjustment for dads, too. Although they don't go through the physical upheaval of actually carrying multiples, from the very first moment dads hear that it's two or more babies instead of one there are plenty of emotional and mental issues they experience that are distinct from what moms—and dads of singleton children—deal with.

Cathy's husband started the twins journey in shock. He hadn't gone with her to the news-breaking sonogram because it was their third pregnancy—they knew the drill by then. His response when Cathy told him over the phone that they were expecting not one but two babies? Dead silence. But several months later, as she was being induced for delivery, he had a panic attack and dropped to the floor. He was rushed to the ER wing of the hospital while Cathy continued with her labor, hoping he would return in time for her to deliver the twins (which he did). This is funny now, especially given the fact that he's six foot six and a former college football player, but it was scary at the time. Cathy thinks her husband took the twin news and bottled it up, something that is much easier for fathers to do than mothers because they are not under-going the physical portion of the pregnancy. (Moms can't really ignore it.) It *is* big news, and there is a scary element, but we suggest Dad try to get his brain around the situation before labor starts, for the good of all involved. Nothing says freak-out like the sound of an offensive lineman fainting.

Many of the moms we surveyed said they survived their twins' hardest stages with the help and support of their husbands or partners, offering comments like "awesome," "lifesaver," and "best husband in the world." It's true: the importance of Dad's role cannot be underestimated for both Mom and the twins. When you're trying to learn how to best support and care for your family given the natural stresses associated with twin parenting (feeding two babies at once, getting two individuals on the same schedule, dealing with two sick children who are up at night), it's much easier with two parents doing the job. To learn from their stories, distill their worries and garner as much practical advice as possible, we interviewed a core group of dads with twins. It was not an easy task to find a date when all the guys could attend; they were all very busy with work and wanted to get home and be with their twins. Even though we offered free beer and bar food, three dads had to bail at the last minute. One was exhausted because his twins had been up screaming the last few nights, another had a splitting headache, and another was under the weather. Moms, it's mentally and physically draining to be a dad of twins, too. Here's what the guys who made it shared.

Our Favorite Dad One-Liners

"Are you sure?"
"We weren't expecting a two-for-one sale."
"We decided to double down."

Five Things Dads of Twins Want Moms to Know

1. If I am on duty, let me do it. Don't look over my shoulder or accuse me of doing it wrong.
2. I miss having sex. I understand that you were restricted on bed rest and for the first several weeks after you had the babies, but I'm still interested.
3. I feel left out. Help me spend quality time with our twins by learning how to manage the chaos.
4. I think you still look hot and your body is amazing for carrying twin babies and producing milk for them.
5. I need downtime, too. My work commute does not count as alone time.

SHOCK AND AWE—IT'S TWINS

The range of reactions reported by dads is really not that wide: those who underwent fertility treatments reported elation at the prospect of having children at all, and something near a sense of relief that it was twins and not triplets, while those who experienced natural twins reported complete and utter disbelief. One dad said, "The possibility never crossed my mind." While the rising twin rate has been fueled largely by the increasing incidence of fertility treatments, advances over the past ten years or so have meant that the rate of triplets (or more) as a result of these treatments has decreased (down 6 percent between 2003 and 2004). Still, twins are a reasonably anticipated outcome, so the shock of it is dimmed a bit. But it can be a hard adjustment to go from aching to have a child to feeling completely thrilled about the prospect of having more than one. Twins are a big responsibility, and even the most welcoming dad might feel intimidated by that challenge, at least initially.

If you're a soon-to-be dad and you're reading this book, chances are the news has already been broken. But rest assured, regardless of the camp you fall into, you are not alone in feeling the rise of your blood pressure and the tightening of your shirt collar.

The important part is that you realize, first and foremost, you have been given the wonderful gift of twins, and second, you need to support the mom-to-be in every way possible as she undergoes the Herculean task of bringing two babies into the world.

HOW DAD CAN GET INVOLVED
IN THE TWIN PREGNANCY

The physical demands of a twin pregnancy are great on a woman, and this is the time when she really needs tons of emotional support, even though it can't relieve all of her symptoms. Some pregnant moms report feeling a division of labor (so to speak) between them and their partner. Medical experts caution extra care during a twin pregnancy. The implication is that things could go "wrong" at any time. That is a lot of mental and emotional pressure added to a pregnant mom's physical discomfort. (The work a soon-to-be dad does in the garage and yard, for instance, might seem pale in comparison to carrying two children in your body!) But alas, nature has made her choice, and women do the baby thing. So the best connection Dad can make to Mom is an emotional one. Dads can get involved and provide support by accompanying Mom on her many sonogram visits, or at least by asking detailed questions about how they went. Seeing your growing babies on the big screen helps relieve dads of some sense of shock and makes it easier to visualize and accept the changes to come. Dads should also ask moms if there's anything they can do to ease the physical discomfort—massage, organization of pillows in bed, or even a foot rub can go a long way!

HOW DADS CAN EASE THE BURDEN
OF BED REST

Twenty-five percent of the women we surveyed were placed on bed rest sometime during their twin pregnancy. One of the dads we interviewed faced the challenge of his wife being placed on hospitalized bed rest during her first pregnancy for five weeks. He would go to work, run home and check the mail, then drive over to the hospital to spend the evening hours with his wife. He said the greatest thing he could provide her with was comfort, the sense that she was not going through this alone. He added that no matter what kind of day he had in the office, it was nothing compared to what she was toughing out. While this is, fortunately, an extreme example, the lesson learned is that dads can show moms that they are in this twins boat together; even if the beginning is a bit choppy, the rest of the cruise should be wonderful. Being a friend and comfort during bed rest is essential, and no one is better qualified to provide that kind of support than Dad. We know of another dad who made weekend nights at home more fun by renting movies and loading up on their favorite munchies. He didn't complain and was there when she needed him. Between the big worries regarding the safety of the babies to the more mundane grind of what needs to get done at home, Mom needs to be reassured daily. If the babies have her belly, Dad needs to have her back.

HOW DADS CAN ADJUST TO
THE TWINS' ARRIVAL

If your twins are your first children, the adjustment to life with young kids is going to override the fact that there are two of them. Changing from a couple to a couple of parents is mind-blowing in and of itself. Sure, it will be more intense for you because you

Married with Twins

Ninety-eight percent of the moms who answered our survey are married. But even the best marriages aren't necessarily twin-proof. Some studies show that parents of twins may be more susceptible to divorce than parents of singletons.

Our own survey highlights some of the twin stress that a marriage faces. When asked about the effect of having twins on their relationships, 55 percent of the moms we surveyed said there is less time for their partner and 20 percent reported increased tension. The official MO for many twin parents is to divide and conquer, which sometimes means Mom and Dad end up spending very little time together. Taking steps to carve out couple time is a big help. When you can, try to run errands as a family or read bedtime stories as a big group. Dads can also help find babysitters and plan date nights. They don't have to be romantic extravaganzas—just a quick meal at the corner diner might be a good way to reconnect and talk about things other than the all-consuming twins. Just going through the motions of getting dressed up and getting in the car together without two little buggers in the backseat makes you feel like you are getting away with something naughty. Adding a little bit of mischief to your marriage can be a good thing! The married-with-twins forecast isn't completely bleak, though, as 10 percent said their relationships are now "twice as nice." Indeed, having children can make a couple feel even more bonded. And for some couples who've dealt with various infertility problems and treatments, having twins leaves them so overjoyed and thankful that they find themselves appreciating their partners more, too.

have twins, but trust us veterans, your head will be spinning so fast there might as well be ten of them!

If your twins come after a singleton or two, you'll notice quite a difference between adding one child versus adding two. The dynamics of your family simply change at an exponential rate with the addition of twins. This can be tough for older siblings and dads; life as you all know it is over. But our focus group of dads tells us that the best way to tackle the change is head-on. Hobbies such as golf and projects such as the roof on the backyard shed are going to have to be put on hold, at least temporarily. The dads we talked to suggest trying to enjoy the here and now—the hard work of twins, and the magic of twins. If your double bundles have recently arrived, you are probably aware that the first twelve weeks or so are a sort of surreal experience as you struggle to assert some kind of control over your life. The next step is to divvy up the work: Mom, Dad, friends, family, and any child care providers you've enlisted to help need to work together to create a safe and loving environment for your twins.

PARENTING TWINS: A PRACTICAL GUIDE FOR DADS FROM DADS

Make yourself available. Just how should a new dad of twins dive in? Many dads, including many first-time dads, even of singletons, feel overwhelmed and ill-equipped to handle newborns. The fear of doing something wrong paralyzes a lot of guys, so they do nothing or think they are being most helpful by staying out of the way. For Christina's husband, watching her rush around the house when their twins first came home from the hospital was like seeing a mini tornado. She was nuts, and he was reluctant to get in her way, so he stood back, waiting to be told what to do. Even though he was eager to participate, Christina misinterpreted his sideline time. Eventually they hashed it out and he was happily put to work. The reality is, dads need to be a part of the madness. The dads we interviewed said that no matter how much or how little your partner actually asks for your help, the best thing you can do is be there to offer it.

These dads pitched in by working out an arrangement at the office to minimize their travel schedules for a few months or taking paternity leave or an extended vacation. Dads can also help by simply working with their partners to establish a routine that plays to their strengths, as well as the twins' routine. For example, Cathy's husband has a fairly regular work schedule, so he can typically arrive home in time for evening care. As a result, the pre-bedtime bathing routine for the twins and their two big brothers is primarily his responsibility. Other dads might be better suited to take charge of the morning routine, allowing Mom to get some extra rest or a few minutes alone to shower and start the day. Later, as your twins get older, it might mean cutting back on hobbies or social activities to attend their weekend soccer games or drive them to and from birthday parties.

Get involved with chores. This means feed babies, change diapers, fold laundry, etc. The moms we surveyed valued the verbal and emotional support as much as the day-to-day help dads provided when the babies arrived. The number one way dads helped was by waking up in the middle of the night to change diapers and feed babies. Even if you are not the baby care type and didn't get too involved with your older children as babies, accept that you are going to have to become involved with your tiny twins. The workload is such that, for the sake of time, safety, and Mom's sanity, two sets of hands are pretty much a requirement.

When Your Dad Friends with Singletons Just Don't Get It

It's like the difference between man-to-man and zone defense. Most dads adjust to life with one child by tag-teaming it with their partners. Even having staggered singletons means having staggered control over kiddie chaos, which is better than no control (what it can feel like when you have twins). Young twins (up to age three at the very least) are extremely demanding. There is just so little time and energy left, hobbies and friends tend to get pushed down to the bottom of the list. This can be hard for friends, especially those with children of their own, to understand. They don't realize it's different with twins. If your buddies are relentlessly teasing you, maybe it is time for a game of hoops or after-work beers. Just do your wife a favor and give her a heads-up, which doesn't mean BlackBerry her from a bar stool.

Be a sounding board and co–decision maker. Work with your partner to make decisions about feeding choices, sleep routines, development, and school. Twins raise some unique parenting challenges: nurturing individual identities and interests, balancing natural bonds and rivalries, and helping child care providers and teachers navigate the twin waters. Getting in sync means a constant dialogue between parents and being supportive of decisions made in your absence.

Bond with your twins your way. Twins have such a special bond that in many cases it's deeper than that of close-in-age siblings. But that does not eliminate the need for interaction with Dad. Remember, your twins still need to engage with you, not just each other, and each individual child needs to establish his or her own relationship with Dad. For Christina's family, the weekend routine often includes father-son trips to Home Depot and then father-daughter grocery store runs. Both twins feel like they are getting alone time with Dad, and Dad is helping the family out by getting chores done.

Twincidentals: **Father-Daughter Bonding** In cases where

Dad is the parent of all girls—the odd man out, so to speak—it might be time for him to put on a tutu and get into the mix. Dads can shoot hoops with girls, teach them to ride bikes and swim, cook them chocolate chip pancakes on Sundays, and learn how to do their hair and who their favorite Disney princess is. In some cases, boy/girl twins mean only one girl child is in the family, possibly with older or younger brothers, and your little darling may need extra TLC from you when the boys get too boyish. Getting in touch with your feminine side will surely be appreciated by your partner.

Contribute financial support. Thirty-four percent of the moms we surveyed reported that finances are the number one thing their partners worry about in relation to their twins. Maybe it's the only thing dads think they can gain some sense of control over, but the stress associated with the traditional role of bread-winner seems to be prevalent. Some of the twin-related financial basics dads can employ to alleviate the stress include joining a warehouse club, setting up 529 plans for college, establishing an emergency fund, and making sure they have enough life insurance. (For tips about finances when twins are in the family, check out our "Money" chapter, page 242.)

Deflect stress. Whether the mom of twins is home or at work, she has a lot on her plate—it's the nature of the job. There are some ways that dads can alleviate the pressure during the first few months of twin parenting: take charge of any older children, allow her to regain her strength and recover physically during the post-partum phase, minimize visits from relatives unless they are expressly requested by your partner, start a Web page with updates on the twins, and kick it up a notch when it comes to regular household jobs. Going forward, when your twins get bigger it's easier to be out and about with twins in tow, so Mom and Dad can alternate breaks, get chores done, and enjoy family outings and activities.

Take safety seriously. In our survey, our moms mentioned the first three months and the eighteen-month-to-three-year range as the hardest times to be twin parents. With the latter, it's mostly because you are double-teamed by active, curious toddlers and preschoolers. During this phase, it's essential that you listen to Mom's concerns about what the twins gravitate toward when it comes to danger, and come clean when they get into twin mis-chief on your watch.

The Babysitter Debate

If the dynamic of your couple is a stay-at-home mom or part-time working mom and full-time working dad, chances are the discussion of whether or not to hire a babysitter has come up. Fifty-three percent of the moms we surveyed classify themselves as stay-at-home moms, and many report having steady paid help. That is costly, but is it a requirement or a luxury? Moms tend to see the help, at various ages and stages, as necessary for safety as well as sanity. Dads who are out of the house at work tend to see it more as a luxury. The twins are expensive enough themselves; it's hard to shell out more cash for babysitting. But it may help to see it as a short-term financial splurge. The payoff could be huge: twins who are safely entertained and a mom who has some downtime or freedom to do errands without two kids in tow. A happier mom means a happier dad.

Tw-ins

and

Outs

5

CHOW TIME

establishing a routine for your twins is key in managing the care and feeding of two tiny babies. That's right—a good routine is a survival skill, and your feeding process is the cornerstone of your routine. You'll begin establishing it whether you decide to nurse, bottle-feed with pumped breast milk or formula, or offer your babies some sort of combination, and your routine will continue to support you as your babies transition to solid food. Sixty-three percent of the moms we surveyed said they had both babies on one feeding schedule during the infant stage, 17 percent did a combination of on-demand and a shared schedule, and 11 percent fed each baby on demand. Only one person admitted she had no schedule at all; in fact, many moms said not establishing a routine sooner was their greatest twin parenting mistake because of its long-lasting chaotic effect. Trust us, you are not your best self under duress, and a routine affords the opportunity to regain some semblance of control over the craziness that is naturally life with twins.

Thrival Tip: Own your routine; don't let your routine own

you. Even if you subscribe to the theory that structure is good for babies, as we both do, you have to be willing to throw the routine out the window as life demands it: when one or both twins are sick, if an invitation comes your way that you can't pass up, even when you just need a break from your own daily grind. If you feel more stress to stay on schedule than you do comfort from the sense of control, it's time to loosen the reins a bit.

Record keeping can be a big help when it comes to establishing and sticking to a routine. Many moms suggested strategies for getting this process started: everything from old-school marble notebooks to new customized electronic mommy systems. While Excel spreadsheets as a parenting approach might seem excessive, when you're a sleep-deprived mother of multiples it's impossible to remember things like "Who ate first on which breast for how long?" and "Who had how many wet and poopy diapers?"

Moms record feedings, diaper changes, food allergies or aversions, pumping schedules, and more to learn to work with their twin babies' natural rhythms. Keeping track of this stuff also makes doctor's visits more productive. One of the favorite modern tools is the Itzbeen, a battery-powered baby care timer that helps new parents remember all the details (see itzbeen.com for more info). All of these tools, especially the do-it-yourself spreadsheet version, might seem like a lot of work at first, but it's easier than feeding and changing each baby twice because you couldn't remember the details (yes, you'll be *that* tired).

THE FIRST MEALS: BREAST-FEEDING

Let there be no doubt: breast milk is the best source of nutrition for newborn babies. The American Academy of Pediatrics (AAP) recognizes that breast-feeding is important for optimal infant and child health and development because of the associated health, nutritional, developmental, psychological, social, economic, and environmental benefits. Breast milk provides antibodies that can help your children fight illness and allergies for years as they grow, and breast-feeding is an unparalleled bonding experience, even when you do it two at a time. Pediatric experts encourage every mother to breast-feed for as long as possible, but having nursed seven babies between us, we know that nursing can be physically, mentally, and emotionally demanding on a mom. It's not something you can take on halfheartedly. It takes commitment, dedication, planning and, in some cases, a willingness to battle through some physical discomfort. But breast milk is so important for your babies, and we know from talking to lots and lots of moms who've done it that it's worth all the effort. And don't forget the bonuses: breast milk is free and there are no bottles to wash!

This ten-step checklist can help you master the art of breast-feeding twins:

1. **Be prepared to stick with it.** Even the most dedicated breast-feeder can run into problems. Talk to your doctor about how to power through physical challenges so you can keep your commitment to yourself and your babies.

2. **Learn the holds.** There's a technique to safely and successfully nursing two babies (see page 78 of this chapter for more details on twin holds).

3. **Teach your babies to latch on.** If there is a qualified professional on hand to help, take advantage. Get over your modesty and allow the hospital nurses to literally put your nipple into the mouths of your babies before you head home.

4. **Stay fed and hydrated.** You absolutely will not be able to nurse two babies if you are not taking care of yourself. Maintaining your strength as the master feeder requires a proactive approach to eating and drinking water (see our "Mom Care" chapter on page 35 for nutritional guidelines for nursing moms).

5. **Create a comfortable environment.** Build your own nursing space: on your bed, on the couch in the family room, in the nursery, wherever you can easily and consistently settle in to feed.

6. **Carve out the time.** Two babies eating every three hours and taking up to an hour each to finish a full feeding can be time-consuming. If you have other things to do, such as care for older children or go to the bathroom every once in a while, you'll need to be organized.

7. **Get support.** Until you get the hang of it, it helps to have four hands to cradle, latch, re-latch and burp your multiples. If you have help, teach them that their primary responsibility is to assist with nursing until you've gotten your strength and your nursing groove.

8. **Maintain your milk supply.** Offering supplemental formula or changing your nursing schedule because of sleeping babies can cause your body to ease up on production. If you want to keep nursing, you have to keep stimulating.

9. **Monitor your babies' weight gain.** It's not always easy to tell just how much your babies are eating when they're nursing. Sometimes this worry can cause you to abandon breast-feeding altogether. Ask your pediatrician if you can come in to weigh your babies periodically (more frequently than for scheduled office visits) to ease your mind and measure your success.

10. **Have realistic expectations.** Nursing twins is not the same as nursing one baby, so cut yourself some slack if you nursed a singleton but have trouble doing it for your twins. Your most heartfelt intentions to do what's best can be shaken by two screaming babies, nursed simultaneously day after day, night after night. Adjust your schedule, get extra help, or supplement with formula to get over the rough spots. The longer you are able to give your babies breast milk, the greater their health benefits.

Cathy nursed her twins for a little over two months; Christina nursed for two weeks and then pumped around the clock for ten more weeks. For both of us, this was a significantly shorter time than we nursed our singleton children. Despite our best intentions, we found the balance between nursing our twins and parenting our older children too much to nurse any longer. Here's the breakdown of how the 68 percent of moms we surveyed who nursed their newborn twins did it:

Thirty-five percent for three months or less
Thirty percent for three to six months
Twenty-four percent for six to twelve months
Eleven percent for more than one year

Mommy Doc: One mom who qualifies for that impressive year-plus category was our own Mommy Doc, Dr. Lori Smith, M.D. Her twins were her firstborn, yet she maintained her pediatric practice and her active pace of life after their birth. We asked her, as a doctor and a fellow mom of twins, what steps she took to set herself up for success.

Here's how she did it:

1. **Positive thinking.** Mommy Doc's nursing frame of mind started before she even entered the labor room. Her mind-set wasn't "We'll see how I feel when it happens." Rather, she went into the delivery mentally prepared to start nursing right away. While pregnant, Mommy Doc consulted the on-line boards of her local Mothers of Multiples club for advice. She learned that, aside from a personal commitment, a special twin nursing pillow (not two regular pillows) is critical to learning correct twin positioning. She brought her pillow to the hospital with her and asked the nurses for support in getting things started. That pillow stuck with her for months at home, at work, and on the go. Many survey moms specifically recommended the EZ-2-Nurse Twins feeding pillow (available at doubleblessings.com or justmultiples.com).

2. **People.** Ask for help often at the hospital from the lactation or nursing staff, as they can teach you and your twins how to master the latch-on. Once home, Mommy Doc was able to count on both her mother and her husband for nursing support. Her husband was given the task of handling the 11:00 P.M. and 3:00 A.M. feedings. Mommy Doc would go to sleep at 8:00 P.M., then he would bring the babies to her, handling all the pre- and post-feeding work involved, or he'd feed them expressed breast milk in bottles.

3. **Process.** You have to teach your babies to latch on and nurse successfully. Developing your own routine so that all three of you are comfortable is important. Mommy Doc recommends latching on one baby, placing a folded baby blanket under that baby's head for support, and then latching on the other. If they latch on well and are fully supported by the breast-feeding pillow and folded blankets under their heads, you

will have free hands to use. Once her babies were a little older and she was strong enough to handle nursing both of them on her own, Mommy Doc found nursing twins while sitting on a couch the easiest. She says, "Organize everything before you sit down: your glass of water or food, something to do"—she even wrote thank-you notes while nursing!—"the phone, etc. Place each baby on the couch in a secure place (not on the edge). Sit down between the two babies, arrange the nursing pillow around you, and then place each baby on top of the pillow and help them latch on." Even though Mommy Doc's son was the stronger nurser, she kept both twins latched and had let down on both breasts. Both twins reaped the benefits of her son's stronger sucking at the same time.

4. **Pumping.** Once back at work (she returned after six months), Mommy Doc scheduled time in her daily calendar for an appointment with her breast pump, but you could also plan to pump during your break time. She says, "I was able to concoct a system so that my hands were free to make phone calls or write at my desk while pumping with an electric pump. Eventually, once the babies were older (closer to one year), I was able to stop pumping during the day and continue to breast-feed in the morning before work and the evening before they went to bed. It was a very manageable and enjoyable experience."

Figuring out your best setup is important on the road to nursing success, and using the right holds can make it easier to nurse the twins longer. The overwhelming majority of breast-feeding mothers we surveyed found that simultaneous nursing became a big time-saver once they got the hang of it. Lactation specialists are experts in all of the methods, so ask for a hands-on demonstration while you're still in the hospital. Some moms even hire lactation consultants to come to their homes for customized help to make the process more comfortable. A specialized twin nursing pillow should also help with all three preferred positions: the cross-cradle, double-clutch, and parallel holds. If possible, have someone help you with extra support pillows as needed.

Cross-cradle hold. Nestle Baby A in your left arm so that her neck rests in the bend of your elbow, her back along your forearm, and her butt in your left hand. Use your right hand to turn her whole body on the side (so her tummy, head, and neck are facing you), tuck her arms out of the way, and raise her to your left breast. Nestle Baby B in your right arm, use your left hand to turn her body to the side and latch her on to your right breast. Their heads should be apart but their legs and feet crisscrossed.

Double-clutch hold. Place Baby A on your left side, supporting your left breast with your right hand and pulling her close with your left arm. Once Baby A is latched on and sucking well, place Baby B on your right side, cupping your right breast with your left hand and pulling Baby B close with your right hand.

Parallel hold. Baby A is in the cradle hold on your left side and Baby B is in the clutch hold on your right side. Their bodies should be lying in the same direction.

For some photos and illustrations of these holds, check out multiplebirthfamilies.com and breastfeeding.com.

Terrific Twinsight:

"I had a hard time getting both babies latched on comfortably. I wound up nursing one while the other got a bottle of formula or pumped milk. At the next feeding, I would switch which baby nursed."

Other moms alternated between simultaneous and individual feedings, depending on the circumstances of their babies and the availability of helping hands. If nursing one baby at a time is better for you, get accustomed to feeding one while comforting the other. The moms we surveyed came up with some creative solutions for keeping the baby who's not currently eating happy and engaged. Some days, it's as easy as keeping the crying baby nearby on the bed or couch while nursing her twin, so you can rub his feet or belly in a gentle soothing manner. Other times, it takes Mom rocking him in his bucket car seat with her foot. The key is, whatever you do, keep both babes close by so you can pacify without having to interrupt the breast-feeding process.

Another complicating factor when it comes to feeding twins is burping. Babies typically want to be burped right after feeding, so there's no waiting around for his or her twin to finish feeding. With twins, the big question is what the heck do you do with the other baby when you're burping one? Don't worry—we moms have devised some ways to divide and conquer:

- Mom can burp one baby over her shoulder with the other baby lying across her lap.
- Mom can pat one baby's back while the infant is resting over her

Twincidentals: Different Appetites

Sometimes one twin takes to nursing (or eating in general) better than the other twin does. Cathy had one son who latched on right away and ate voraciously and agreeably during every feeding, while his twin never really got the hang of latching on and, in fact, was not that interested in food no matter how it was offered to him. She tried nursing the less interested twin at each feeding; sometimes there were tears (hers and his) and screams (his) and other times it worked. This can be challenging, especially when they are infants and you're trying to take an egalitarian approach to parenting. Don't let it get you down. Rather, focus on your priority: to help your babies thrive. If that means nursing exclusively for one and supplementing for the other, you're not playing favorites, you're being flexible.

knees, with the other baby reclining at an upright angle (with pillow support) next to her on the couch.

- Mom can pump the legs of one baby on the bed or couch with the other nearby.

GETTING PUMPED

Keeping up your milk supply is critical to long-lasting nursing success. Sometimes when you miss a feeding for whatever reason (babies start to sleep for longer stretches and you skip a feeding, you need to be away from the babies to attend to other commitments such as older children or work, or you are just exhausted and need to sleep and hand off a bottle-feeding to another adult) your milk supply can begin to wane. Rather than relying on your babies, the best way to manage your supply is to pump, as did 68 percent of the survey moms who offered their babies breast milk. Because they are moms of twins, no small handheld pump would do, so most used an electric or even hospital-grade pump to get that milk out.

According to Mommy Doc, expressed (pumped) breast milk offers no less benefit to your babies than milk nursed right from your breasts. Plus it can be frozen or stored in the fridge, then put in bottles for feeding by you or another capable caretaker (which could mean sleep for you!). A pumping routine affords moms more control over their milk supply. As one mom described it, pumping extended the length of time she was able to offer her babies her "special momma milk."

BOTTLE-FEEDING: MORE FLEXIBILITY FOR MOM

The plastic is coming! The plastic is coming! We were floored by all the plastic and rubber that took over our kitchens when we had

Pumping Tips

- **Make mommy cocktails.** Mix just-expressed milk with formula (the total amount of ounces should equal your pediatrician's recommendation) and serve it to babies in bottles. You might gain some peace of mind when you see how much breast milk your babies are drinking.
- **Tolerate midnight madness.** The secret of maintaining your milk supply is constant stimulation. Consider setting an alarm to wake up in the middle of the night and express milk, the way Christina and some survey moms did, however insane that may seem. Before you go to bed for the night, make sure you have everything you need nearby to pump and store the milk (mini-fridge or a cooler with an ice pack and enough clean storage containers for the breast milk).

our twins. Think about it: most newborns eat approximately every three hours, so that's at least eight bottles per day, multiplied by two (or more).

Some of the same strategies that work for breast-feeding two infants can apply when you're bottle-feeding. Absent a second set of hands, you can use pillows, arranged at gentle angles, to give your babies' heads a lift, to prevent them from rolling onto the floor, and to be able to reach both of them while controlling the bottles. You'll need to find a comfortable setting and arrange your pillows (many moms we surveyed used two Boppy pillows) to safely and securely feed your twins.

Bottle-feeding multiples also comes with its own set of issues. One issue is that even when things go smoothly, eight or more bottles a day can make you feel like you are working an assembly line. The upside of the process is that you can manage it. If you hand-wash the bottles, you may get into this groove: feed babies, burp, change, let them play, wash bottles, put on dish-drying rack. At the end of the night, no matter how tired you are, it helps to take all your clean bottles and refill them with the next day's supply of formula or pumped milk (63 percent of survey moms prepared bottles ahead of time to make things easier on themselves). One mom said she'd make a pitcher of formula instead of taking up room in the fridge with eight or more pre-made bottles. Other moms run the bottles through the dishwasher and refill them early in the mornings.

Twin Set Confidential: Many of the moms we surveyed said they utilized self-feeding bottles and bottle props to manage bottle-feeding two babies simultaneously. The AAP does not support these products primarily because of associated choking risks. (Clearly, babies should never be left unattended, not even for a second, with liquid food pouring into them from a bottle.) Although not recommended by doctors, the Podee Hands-Free Baby Bottle was a favorite with many survey moms. Cathy used foam bottle props (which she found at greatbabyproducts.com) to help her feed her twins. She would sit in between her guys while they were in bucket car seats or bouncy seats and hold up the props. She relied on this technique until her twins were around six months and could hold their own bottles. The bottom line: self-feeding bottles and props can be very helpful, but you should use them with caution if you choose to do so.

A second issue, even for us (combination breast- and bottle-feeders), was the shocking quantity—and cost—of formula we needed to tank up our little ones. We became fanatical formula-coupon hunters. We bought powdered formula at a local whole-sale club, and Christina drove twenty-five miles north to a big baby store that sold liquid formula for $4 less a case than she could get locally. She'd buy at least ten cases at a time to make it worth the gas money (for more money-saving tips, check out our "Money" chapter, page 242).

A third issue is keeping track of which bottle belongs to which twin. To alleviate confusion, you can write their names or initials on their bottles with a Sharpie (heads-up: the ink may get washed off the bottle after a while, and you may need to relabel the bottles regularly). Or you can buy the same brand of bottles in different colors or with different color bottle rings. Christina bought two of Gerber's rainbow-colored six-packs of bottles and used the blue, green, and purple ones for her son, and the red, orange, and hot-pink ones for her daughter. Or you can even buy each twin a different brand of bottle, as Cathy did.

STRAPPED IN:
BABY TWINS TRANSITION TO FOOD

Around six months of age, we introduced our babies to food. This was an exciting time for us: our babies began to sit upright in high chairs, wear plastic bibs, and eat mush (aka baby cereal). Then they moved toward actual food such as strained fruits and veggies, and even crackers. Near their first birthdays, we switched from bottles and formula to milk and cups. We were thrilled to stop spending a small fortune on formula and just include more milk in our grocery hauls. Day by day, we added more and more food to our twins' growing menus: chopped meat, cheese, yogurt, eggs, tiny pieces of fruit and veggies. Watching them enjoy their independence and explore new tastes and textures provided priceless parenting moments.

Twincidentals: **To Have and Two to Hold** If you simultaneously bottle-feed your twins, this means they may not be held as often as if you fed them one at a time. You can create more opportunities for closeness by alternating between simultaneous feedings and one-at-a-time feedings, or you can have some helpers come over to hold and feed one baby, so you can do the same with the other.

A Word About Twins and High Chairs

There's no getting around it: you'll need two of these. Buying the chairs that are best for your family dynamic is important. Some purchase considerations include cost, convenience, versatility, and space constraints. If your budget and space are tight, hold off on buying high chairs until you really need them. When your twins start cereal, around 4–6 months, they might be too little for a high chair, so you can feed them in their bouncy or car seats or strollers. For safety's sake, baby twins need the security of high chairs with a five-point harness.

Yet, despite the undeniable mealtime cuteness, feeding twins can leave you feeling as if all you do is prepare, serve, and clean up the mess from food. Trust us, we still spend a lot of time in the kitchen, and more than we care to account for on our hands and knees picking up Cheerios. (And the food grind is directly related to the laundry grind. See our "Clean Kids" chapter, page 121.)

FIVE SECRETS OF TRANSITIONING TO "REAL FOOD"

1. **Manage your equipment.** You may not be able to predict how cooperatively your twins will eat each day, but you can help things run more smoothly by doing some advance work. Make sure you have enough clean bowls and spoons, and regularly de-crud the high chairs (see our "Clean Kids" chapter, page 121, for tips on keeping high chairs clean). To save space, get a couple of stackable plastic bowls with travel lids for each twin. Sometimes the lids get warped in the dishwasher, so you may want to hand-wash them. Many moms we surveyed used color-coding systems to better manage the feeding process, because it can be tough to remember who is eating from which bowl of mashed banana when they are both visibly hungry and excited.

Twincidentals: The Squeaky Wheel

Sometimes it's just easier on everyone when the crying twin is fed first, certainly during the early, messy months of feeding. This can mean that the same child is left waiting for bottle, cereal, and food over and over again. The challenge is making sure this doesn't carry over to all areas of behavior, so one twin is unintentionally relegated to second place. To balance things out, you can give the less anxious eater first dibs on bath time. And be sure to feed her first when her more vocal sister is quiet for a change at mealtime.

2. **Create personal space for each twin.** At mealtime, when both twins are literally starved for your undivided attention, closeness is not necessarily the best environment. Too-close twins tend to steal food from each other's high chair trays and start food fights. To avoid this, keep a safe distance between them at meals and foster the intimacy between siblings at a more relaxed time, such as during bedtime stories.

When Twins Throw Their Food

Sometimes all it takes is one twin to lob a banana slice over to his twin's high chair, and a full-fledged food fight breaks out. To avoid this mutiny, limit the amount of food you put in front of your twins, waiting until they eat what's in front of them before you give them more. You can also put a good distance between their chairs while they are eating, and separate them even more if they don't act nicely. You can also avoid serving food that you'll resent cleaning up (Christina's son loves rice, but she only makes it once every couple of weeks). If one or both twins ignore your attempts to keep them in line, you can clean them off and remove them from the kitchen (and your presence, so they won't be getting your attention). Put the food thrower(s) in a safe place (the play yard, the crib) so you'll all get a chance to calm down.

3. **Master in-sync feeding.** It's clumsy to feed two hungry babies by using two hands to scoop up food from two bowls using two spoons. Our favorite service method: strap the babies into their seats, serve each something to nosh on (a hard roll or mini bagel), then seat yourself in the middle on a chair. Alternate feeding one spoonful at a time to each twin.

4. **Banish germophobia.** Fear not, you can get away with rewashing one or two baby spoons all day. In fact, 63 percent of moms surveyed confess that they regularly feed both babies from the same spoon (unless one is sick, of course). The thinking is that the twins slobber all over the same toys and suck on each other's hands and feet, so why not share a spoon and make feeding simpler for Mom? The key is knowing *when* to worry about germs—and if they both seem relatively healthy, it's not during regular daily feedings.

5. **Plan your baby food.** Since Cathy had two older boys to cook for every day, she found it easier to make baby food alongside the rest of the family's meal, rather than use the jarred stuff. For Christina, the thought of putting a banana and mango in a ricer or mini food processor in addition to cooking for the rest of her bunch was overwhelming, so she stuck with the jars. Either way, you have to make space in your freezer, fridge, and pantry, and you have to make sure you have adequate supplies on hand. Cathy got into the habit of shopping at the organic produce store or local farmers' market once a week. She'd prepare the food when she was already in the kitchen prepping other meals. She'd serve some to her twin boys immediately and save the rest in labeled storage containers in the fridge for the next day or two. Christina, with coupons in hand, loaded up for at least a couple of weeks. Think about it—at least six jars a day for seven days is forty-two jars! If babies have different preferences, it can get confusing, so make a list and take it with you.

"Picky eating" and food jags (periods when your child will eat only a limited variety of foods) are common complaints among parents of toddlers. According to nutritionist Soniyu Perl, these ideas can help you make mealtime more enjoyable:

- Offer a variety of wholesome, nutritious foods, including foods that you know each child likes.
- Allow each twin to choose, but if one decides to eat nothing, respect her choice—even if her twin is scarfing his meal down. She'll make up for it at the next meal or the next day.

Although frustrating, picky eating is often a normal stage of development and won't last forever. However, if your toddler is not gaining sufficient weight, discuss your concerns with your pediatrician.

As your twins get more comfortable with "real food," you'll want to keep exposing them to new tastes and expanding your menu options. Perl shares her own mom-tested tips for getting twins excited about new foods:

Twincidentals: **Two Choosy Eaters** Despite the temptation to handle your twins as one unit, they will continually remind you that they are individuals—which means separate likes and dislikes when it comes to food. At different ages and stages, this manifests itself in different ways: one twin likes rice cereal, while the other wants oatmeal; you have one fruit gal, while her twin is all about the veggies. Moms repeatedly told us that they want to indulge their twins' individuality in the kitchen, but it's just not practical to do it at every meal.

Get them involved. Let your twins choose the food or help make it; select one new fruit or vegetable each week when you go shopping.

Make it fun. Put vegetables on kabobs or on top of a favorite food such as pizza; make a veggie face on the plate; serve vegetables with dip such as yogurt, low-fat salad dressing, or even peanut butter.

Take them to the source. Plan an outing to an orchard or berry farm.

Be a good role model. If you're eating lots of junk or skip meals, you can't expect your kids to eat properly. Make an effort to eat whole grains, fruits, and vegetables when you're hungry, and chances are that eventually your twins will, too. (Check out our "Mom Care" chapter, page 35, for Perl's healthy eating tips for you.)

Keep at it. Above all, don't give up. Your twins will learn to try and like a variety of foods, but only if they're offered. Perl says it can take eight to twelve exposures for a child to taste the food, let alone like it, so don't give up after the first try.

FREE AT LAST: TODDLER TWINS LEAVE THE HIGH CHAIR

All good things must come to an end. For moms of multiples, it's a huge bummer when the twins revolt against being strapped in high chairs or booster seats at mealtime. The result: two unfettered kids who can slip off their chairs in the middle of a meal to pet the dog with sauce-covered hands, or two kids who take three bites of the meal you took forty-three minutes to prepare, declare they're full, and run toward the play area. Just how do moms of twins get the best out of their two-to-five-year-olds before, during, and after mealtime? Taste this advice for yourself.

Speak preschoolese. To encourage our toddlers to follow instructions, we looked toward our kids' nursery school teachers—virtual mothers of multiples—to observe how they get a group of same-age kids to cooperate at snack time. You can use phrases from the classroom at home. For example, "Arms up if you can hear me. Okay, good. Now let's see who can eat without spilling today."

Give them jobs. Once your twins are around three years old, you can give them each a simple mealtime task at home. For instance, one can fold napkins and the other can place spoons on them. It makes twins feel good to work together, which often translates into better mealtime behavior.

Cleanup Tools Twins Can Use

Wipes. Keep them on the kitchen counter, within your reach. Your twins may not be babies anymore, but they could still benefit from the magic of wipes. They can clean up their own juice-box spills before the counter gets super sticky. And they can start erasing signs of pizza and chocolate ice cream on their own hands and faces.

Hand vacs. These are light and simple enough for a three-year-old to use to suck up just-spilled cereal. Have one twin vacuum first, then the other mop (see below).

Mops with floor wipes. These mops often require some assembly, which means you can take out one piece and make the mop shorter to suit your twins' heights.

A Double Serving: Two Twin-Friendly Recipes

We're both suckers for shortcuts when it comes to cooking for and feeding our children. Our favorite meals are easy to prepare and long-lasting (meaning tasty leftovers). Here are each of our favorite recipes that fit the bill.

Christina's Chicken Soup

1 medium white or yellow onion
2 tablespoons olive oil
3 celery stalks
2 cups baby carrots
2–3 cups cooked chicken breast
10–12 cups chicken stock
2 bay leaves
$1/2$ lb pasta
Salt and pepper to taste

Dice the onion and sauté it in olive oil with a dash of salt and pepper on a low flame. While the onion turns clear, chop the celery stalks and carrots into bite-size pieces. Dump them in the pot with the onions and give them a stir. Let the veggies cook for about 5 minutes while you chop up the chicken. Add the chicken stock to the pot and toss the cut chicken in. Throw in the bay leaves and let the soup come to a boil. After it boils, reduce heat and let it simmer until the veggies are soft. Season with salt and pepper. While it cooks, get a second pot filled with water and a dash of salt. Bring that pot to a boil and put your favorite noodles or small pasta in it. Cook the pasta according to the box directions. When your soup is cooked and you are ready to serve, put the pasta in your soup bowls first, then pour the soupy part on top. This way the pasta doesn't get mushy. You can double the batch and freeze half for a later date. Enjoy!

Cathy's Comfort Food

1 whole chicken
Kosher salt and white pepper
Enough sweet potatoes to feed your bunch
Orange juice
French green beans (the skinny kind)

Lightly season the chicken with salt and pepper and place in a roasting pan. Put a small amount of water in the bottom of the roasting pan, cover the meat with foil, and bake at about 325 degrees approximately 20 minutes per pound. Meanwhile, prick the sweet potatoes with a fork, wrap in foil, and bake them until they are soft (about an hour). When they are ready, mash them up with a fork and blend in a dash of orange juice for a sweet touch. Boil a small amount of water, then blanch the green beans for about ten seconds. Run cold water over them so they stay crisp, then plate and serve. All four of Cathy's kids love this meal. It's simple, easy to manage, and healthy. The only downside: multiple dishes to clean.

6

SLEEP STRATEGIES

I f you're reading this at two in the morning while listening to your newborns cry in stereo, the fact that you *will* get a full night's sleep again may seem impossible. Multiple newborns are very demanding physically, mentally, and emotionally. The first few weeks are especially brutal. That's because you need sleep to recover from carrying and delivering two babies—and at the same time, their demands require you to have increased energy, strength, and patience. Yet you're getting a fraction of the rest you need *because* you have two newborn babies who don't sleep when you want them to. Our survey revealed that almost half (44 percent) of the moms felt that sleep deprivation was the hardest hurdle to overcome after the birth of their twins. Many of them reported that "lack of sleep" was Dad's biggest worry, too. Being chronically tired might motivate you to take some action to return to a sane family sleep schedule.

FIVE WAYS TO GET SOME SLEEP

1. **Set realistic goals.** Instead of lamenting the eight hours of sleep you used to get, learn to be happy with a five-hour chunk for a while. Many of the moms of twins we know said they felt they could handle things getting five hours of sleep per night for the first few months of their twins' lives. Of course, some nights you'll get more, some less. But an average of five hours a night is a good and realistic aim.

2. **Take it when you can get it.** Our survey respondents kept repeating this valuable piece of advice: sleep when the babies sleep. This means thinking of your bedtime in a new light. Instead of falling asleep after leisurely watching a *Law & Order* rerun at ten, you may have to make your new, temporary bedtime much earlier or much later. And if the only way for you to get anything close to five hours of sleep is by handing the babies off to your husband and sleeping from, say, 8:00 P.M. to 1:00 A.M., then off those babies go. One mom from our survey said, "Typically, my sleep time was from 7:00 P.M. to 11:00 P.M. My husband had that shift—he was up anyway. If the girls were still sleeping at 11:00, I could possibly catch more sleep for another hour or two if I was lucky."

3. **Do whatever it takes.** You may need to rely on creative methods to get your twins to fall and stay asleep. For example, Baby A may sleep better in the car seat and Baby B may prefer the Moses basket. Don't worry if they aren't snoozing in the bassinets or cribs the way you'd thought they would. There are several reasons why new babies may sleep better in an upright position in a car seat or baby swing (maybe they like being rocked to sleep or they have reflux or nasal congestion). Other babies may prefer the snug and cozy feeling that a Moses basket offers. Almost 70 percent of our moms said their twins regularly slept in car seats, Moses baskets, and swings during the first six weeks at home. You can train your twins to sleep comfortably in more traditional sleep destinations in

a couple of weeks, when you are feeling more up for the challenge. But for now, you can kick into survival mode to rest and regain some strength.

4. **Find and train good help.** Unfortunately, there are very few people you can ask to take over feeding two newborns late at night or in the wee hours. Although your partner may be extremely supportive and helpful with middle-of-the-night care, the reality is that eventually he may need to catch up on his sleep because he's got to function at work the next day. Even if your mom or mother-in-law is ready and willing to do a middle-of-the-night feeding shift, she might not be physically able to manage the two babies at that odd hour or to recover the next day.

   Many moms of multiples are recovering from a C-section and can't lift the babies for a few weeks. Others have older kids who need to be driven to school or other activities in the morning and afternoon. Carpooling isn't always a feasible option, and it's a dangerous undertaking to get behind the wheel when you are chronically sleep-deprived. For some of these moms of twins, the need to get the middle-of-the-night support that a paid professional such as a baby nurse can offer is more of a necessity than a luxury (for more information about your child care options, see our "Good Help" chapter, page 169).

   If the cost of a baby nurse is prohibitive or if you are struggling to find a good one, consider padding your daylight hours with help instead—the point being that if you can hand off just one feeding session to catch a nap during the day, you'll have more stamina during the toughest of nights. It's weird to have your guests come over so you can head to the basement for some slumber instead of chatting. But you can reconnect with your friends and family when your life resumes some degree of normalcy.

5. **Be patient.** We know from parenting our older singletons that time and the maturation of your babies' bodies may be your biggest

A Good Night's Rest

If you want hard proof, here's when the twins of our survey moms finally rested for five consecutive hours or more:

Seven percent said at less than ten weeks (Cathy's experience)

Twenty-two percent said between ten and twelve weeks (Christina's experience)

Forty-one percent said between three and six months

Nineteen percent said six months to one year

Seven percent said more than one year

ally in the quest for more sleep. For all kids, something eventually clicks in their biological and neurological development that enables them to sleep more soundly in longer stretches. With twins, this can mean that one is ready to sleep through the night way before the other, which won't quite alleviate your middle-of-the-night responsibilities. But the other twin will soon be ready for longer sleeps, too. We promise: it happens.

Twincidentals: The Darkest Hours It is extremely diffi-

cult to overcome the challenge of feeling exhausted and alone in the middle of the night as you try to comfort two screaming infants. You may feel frustrated that you're not able to hold and soothe both babies simultaneously. Plus, you may be convinced that you're the only person awake at this ridiculous hour. Exhaustion can drive you to your toughest times: sitting on the floor in the dark crying, locking yourself in the bathroom so you can't hear the babies' howling, even screaming profanities at your wailing newborn babies. It is imperative that you take steps to avoid these low points or at least manage those lonely nights.

Christina wouldn't have made it through those first few weeks had she not had her husband, mother, father, and sister to confide in during daylight hours. Cathy was comforted by caring family and had friends who'd just been through infant twin boot camp. If you don't have friends with twins, there are lots of things you can do to help yourself get in a better frame of mind. You can pray for patience, meditate and take deep breaths, wake your husband for help, ask your mother to come back for another week, or hire a baby nurse for a couple of nights a week. Do what you have to do to stay healthy for yourself and your babies. And definitely talk to your doctor about your physical and emotional struggles and symptoms. (For more information on sleep deprivation and PPD, read our "Mom Care" chapter, page 35.)

INFANT TWINS *CAN* SLEEP THROUGH THE NIGHT

Many of our survey moms told us that getting their twins to sleep through the night was their biggest parenting success. After your babies are a few weeks old and you've done whatever it takes to get some rest so you can begin to recover physically and emotionally from your delivery, you may want to consider being a little more proactive about where and when your babies sleep.

When our babies were about three weeks old, we had nursing, pumping, and bottle-feeding sorted out, and had gotten enough shut-eye to feel more human. We decided it was time to start helping our twins sleep through the night, because they certainly couldn't sleep in their car seats or Moses baskets or strollers forever. It was essential to our thrival to assert more control than these temporary solutions offered, and we were scared that it'd be too hard to undo certain sleep habits, such as being rocked to sleep, down the road.

Lessons Learned: What Desperate Moms Regret Doing to Get their Babies to Sleep

We've both cracked under the pressure and broken our own sleep training rules, especially when we were at the mercy of our twins' illnesses or teething. Just breaking a rule once won't create a problematic sleep habit. But a few nights in a row can create sleep habits that become an issue down the road. Some moms confessed their own twin sleep mistakes:

- "Coddling my daughter at night to get her to sleep because she had colic. Now my son [her twin] goes to sleep within fifteen minutes of being put to bed and my daughter can take two hours!"
- "Letting them sleep in our bed when they wake up in the middle of the night."
- "Rocking them to sleep and not letting them fall asleep in their cribs."

Be prepared—teaching babies good sleep habits is not for the faint of heart. Although these techniques can help your babies fall asleep by themselves, sleep on a more predictable schedule, and stay asleep for longer stretches of time, there are moments of letting one or both babies cry it out that can torture you. But you can put your own spin on a certain technique and set your own limits to make the process less painful (say, five to ten minutes of crying a night before you go in to comfort the baby or babies, instead of increasing the duration of crying each night by five minutes as the well-known Ferber sleep method suggests).

Terrific Twinsight: "Do what works for you and your family. There is no single right way. Every set of multiples is different and has different challenges. Being a mom of twins or being a mom period is hard."

Three Sleep Books That Can Help You

Like us, many of our survey respondents hit the books to see what the experts had to say about helping infants learn to snooze. Here are the most-cited sleep strategies.

On Becoming Baby Wise by Gary Ezzo and Robert Bucknam, fourth ed. (Parent-Wise Solutions, 2006)

A review from our survey: "Read the book *Baby Wise*. People think it's a controversial book. But I took what I needed from it. It helped me devise a schedule for me and my babies. And it helped me learn how to get them to sleep through the night by eight weeks old."

Pros: Our personal favorite, our survey's most endorsed sleep book, and the only one written by a parent of triplets. One mom from our survey thinks it was so effective she said, "I wish I had used *Baby Wise* sooner." And another said, "I have followed *Baby Wise* with all five of my kids. I love this book. It helped me develop a routine, which is more than a schedule, and that made me feel more effective in understanding and meeting my children's needs." During the day, we stuck like glue to the suggested eat-play-sleep cycle. Babies would be fed, burped, and then engaged in some playful activity ("Old MacDonald" on our laps, side-by-side activity mats, or rotating play stations). We put our babies to sleep when they'd had enough activity (they'd cry, yawn, or rub their eyes); they were not fed to sleep, a common temptation.

Cons: The controversy comes because the book suggests that you let your babies learn to fall asleep by comforting themselves. This skill can take a while for babies to master, so for most there is some crying, which is hard for any mom to take. Also, this method required us to be very structured during the course of the day, which was not easy with other kids to care for as well.

Secrets of the Baby Whisperer by Tracy Hogg (Ballantine Books, 2005)

A review from our survey: "Using the easy method from *The Baby Whisperer* was the best twin parenting advice I got. It really helped me get them on a schedule."

Pros: The book's intention is to teach parents how to decipher the meaning of their babies' different cries. If you can tell if your baby is tired, hungry, or in distress, then you know how to help your baby stop crying. It also offers hope that you can undo bad sleep habits in three days. The book focuses on an eat-play-sleep routine, which is similar to other sleep strategies. The text is very anecdotal and has a can-do attitude.

Cons: It may be hard to tell why each baby is crying if they are both crying at the same time, which may happen frequently. The book suggests a staggered feeding schedule for moms of twins. She acknowledges that this gives Mom about thirty minutes of downtime before the next feeding cycle, but it doesn't offer much of a break if you have other kids to care for.

Healthy Sleep Habits, Happy Child by Marc Weissbluth, M.D. (Ballantine Books, 2005)

A review from our survey: "This was my favorite book after the boys were born."

Pros: There's something reassuring about learning sleep habits from a pediatrician and father of four. The author is sympathetic toward parents of twins and devotes a few pages to them in the back of the book. As with much information in the book, the twin section is largely anecdotal—from parents who have solved their kids' sleep problems.

Cons: The author talked to several parents at a support group for parents of twins and discovered that for them to get their twins on the same sleep routine they would often wake the good sleeper from a nap to keep pace with the bad sleeper. He says that consequently the bad sleeper runs the risk of being overtired for being up too long. But he doesn't really offer any detailed solutions to avoid this conflict, other than keeping a sleep log to observe their nap time and wakeful behaviors to discover how to strike a better compromise.

THREE STEPS TO GETTING YOUR BABIES TO SLEEP

The bottom line: there is no single right way of doing things when it comes to the care of your twins. But if you're interested in taking charge of your babies' sleep habits, we came up with three steps—an amalgamation of popular sleep strategies, our own expertise, and the wisdom revealed by our survey respondents. You can tailor them to the reality of your own family. Be willing to cut yourself some slack and adjust your approach as needed.

1. **Stick to the routine.** Establishing a routine or a regular order for doing things is a great way to achieve a baseline level of sanity in the

household. Your "right routine" is personal and should be malleable, but by implementing a consistent order (e.g., eating, sleeping, changing, bathing) you begin to create a predictable rhythm or pattern. Unlike a schedule, a routine is not clock-focused. It's more like an outline for your day. It's comforting to have a routine when things go kaflooey (which happens when one or both twins are sick, teething, or just being difficult). One mom acknowledges the peace of mind a routine can bring: "Everything is a phase. If they aren't sleeping or eating well, just stick with the same routine, and in a few days it will correct itself."

Instead of being a slave to your routine, your routine should empower you: soon your babies recognize bath time as the signal that bedtime is approaching. Now it's easier to get them to sleep. A routine also makes it easier for someone else to step in and follow your procedures, and it allows you to weave in necessary absences to tend to other responsibilities, such as a job or older children, or to get in a nap when you're feeling particularly worn down. You can keep your twins on a good routine for months and years. See page 103 for two sample routines you can try with your infant twins. One of our moms sees the payoff: "By sticking with it, ours are fifteen months, take two 2-hour naps a day, go to bed at 7:00 P.M., and wake up at 7:15 A.M. Not bad!"

2. **Swaddle your twins.** Twins are used to and comforted by close quarters. During those beginning weeks, they really need you to simulate the tight and warm feeling of being together in your womb by swaddling each of them individually in a soft blanket. There are a few different ways to wrap a baby tightly in a blanket, and the nurses in the maternity ward can show you how they like to do it. If possible, practice under their supervision, so they can give you pointers. Your husband should practice there as well. If you leave the hospital feeling as if neither of you has quite mastered swaddling

Twin Set Confidential: We know that your pediatrician probably won't recommend that you use a sleep positioner (a washable, cloth-covered foam wedge that you can Velcro to a cloth mat to help hold a baby in place on her side or back) because the American Academy of Pediatrics considers them a SIDS risk. But some moms from our survey used them anyway, to keep their twins from disturbing each other while sleeping in the same crib. Christina, not aware that the AAP didn't recommend them, used sleep positioners for a couple of weeks, too. She never talked to her pediatrician about them. She just felt like her twins liked the extra-snug feeling that the positioners, in addition to a good swaddle, provided because they were used to being cozied up in her belly. During the time her babies were in positioners, they slept in their bassinets and portable cribs right by her bed. Perhaps if she'd known about the SIDS risk, she wouldn't have used the positioners.

yet, you can ask the nurses at your pediatrician's office for tips and keep practicing at home. Also, there are swaddling blankets sold that make it easier to wrap babies and keep them snug safer and longer. We found great swaddling blankets at lovingbabyinc.com, Sleepsacks at halosleep.com, and SwaddleMe adjustable infant wraps at kiddopotamus.com.

3. **Find sleeping arrangements that your twins like.** Size, maturity, and personal preferences all factor into the logistical decisions around where your babies will sleep most comfortably. Some babies like having their twin close by, while others have been waiting a long time for some elbow room. If your newborn twins like sleeping in the same crib, as 75 percent of the moms we surveyed said theirs did, then consider two swaddled babies placed side by side in a bassinet or cradle. A good swaddle keeps arms and legs

from flailing and waking up the other twin. The physical proximity encourages them to start dealing with (and eventually ignoring) each other's sleep idiosyncrasies (crying, snoring, loud thumb sucking). One mom from our survey observed: "They slept so much better knowing the other was close. Even if one was screaming, the other would sleep right through. Just knowing she was close was enough." You can also place two swaddled babies head to head in the crib. Babies can't kick each other in this position but can coo and gurgle each other to sleep. Typically, kicking out of tight swaddling happens around eight weeks of age. Then, placing them next to each other without swaddling lets them seek each other out for co-soothing.

TWO TYPES OF TWIN ROUTINES: SYNCHRONIZED OR STAGGERED

Synchronized

Twins are fed at the same time (either nursed or bottle-fed), changed, given playtime together, and then put to sleep together. A few lucky moms of identicals reported that their twins put themselves on a synchronized routine without much prodding from Mom.

Pros: *Once Mom works out the best way to feed both twins together, it's a nice way for the twins to bond with Mom as a team. This routine may ultimately take less time than a staggered routine and allow Mom to spend time with other kids or deal with other responsibilities or take a nap!*

Cons: It can be tricky for some moms to nurse babies simultaneously, even with the right nursing pillow. It also takes time to get the hang of bottle-feeding two babies at once. This method also requires waking a sleeping baby for the sake of the routine, which

Sleep Problem Solving

If your twins aren't the best bunkmates, consider these approaches.

- **Sleeping in separate cribs in the same room.** Bigger newborns (such as Cathy's, weights 6 pounds 10 ounces and 7 pounds 9 ounces) appreciate the space to stretch and yawn without making someone else cry. But it's not easy making space in a room for two cribs. Sometimes the decision is made before you get home from the hospital. As one mom said, "I wanted them to sleep in the same crib, but the hospital wouldn't allow it. So once we came home, they slept in their own Pack 'n Play and then moved to their own cribs." One mom's motivation early on was to avoid the emotional drama involved with separating twins later: "I still have mixed feelings about my decision. I hear other moms of twins talking about co-sleeping, and as cuddly as that sounds, I don't think I could deal with breaking them up as they got older. I separated them from the beginning, but I think they are just as close as other twins that co-slept."

- **Sleeping alone in different rooms.** They definitely won't bother each other this way, but it doesn't seem to be a practical parenting solution. What do you do if they are both crying at the same time? Run from room to room? Plus, you may not have enough "official" bedrooms to sleep two kids separately. If this is your only option, consider converting an office or dining room into a makeshift bedroom. If possible, you may want to wait until the twins are toddlers or older to separate them into different bedrooms. It's often harder to get twin toddlers to fall asleep than twin babies because toddlers want to play. One mom from our survey agrees: "As they have gotten older, they do wake each other up and sometimes keep each other up before going to sleep by playing, laughing, and jumping on the bed."

75 percent of the moms we surveyed say they have done to keep their multiples in sync.

A Synchronized Routine

- **Early morning wake-up.** Start the routine for the day after Twin A wakes up. Wake up Twin B, then feed them together, burp them, and change them. Then put them right back down to sleep

Twincidentals: **One Early Riser** Many of our moms are convinced that one of their twins regularly wakes up before the other to ensure some alone time with Mom or Dad. When you finally figure out that this twin isn't out to ruin your morning but is just trying to carve out some space without his or her twin around, it's kind of adorable. Enjoy the one-on-one time. You'll be waking both of them up for middle school before you know it. Christina's twins seem to take turns, week by week, at who gets up first to hang with Mom in the wee hours. But she can tell they delight in being the first up (asking with a smile, "Mom, where's everyone?") and having her complete attention. That is, after she has a couple of sips of coffee.

for the first nap of the day. (Our babies slept most soundly during these hours.) Take the opportunity to sleep, talk to your husband, or get older children ready and off to school.

- **Midmorning wake-up and tandem feeding.** This is when the day really starts. Sometimes you'll need to wake a sleeping baby in order to remain on a synchronized schedule. After feeding, babies should be engaged with some activity while strapped safely into swings or bouncy seats (a good opportunity for you to shower or eat breakfast).

- **Lunchtime double feed, followed by a sponge bath.** This helps wash away the morning grime (including breakfast) and serves as a sleep signal to set the stage for a quality nap.

- **Late afternoon wake-up and double feed, followed by some kind of outing** such as taking a walk or running an errand. Some babies take another short snooze just before dinner (which might give you an hour to feed other children). If your twins are fighting this late afternoon nap, do your best to keep babies engaged and active. Bouncy seats, swings, and play mats are good options for keeping the twins busy. Older siblings can also provide entertainment.

- **Dinnertime double feed and bath.** After they are fed each evening, you can send the twins a strong signal that you're beginning the process of getting them ready to go down for the night. Strip both babies down to their diapers and place them on their backs in the crib with all the lights on. One by one, give baths followed by a rubdown. Yes, the waiting baby is typically crying, but soothing sounds such as classical music from a portable CD player or the Fisher-Price aquarium can help. One tip: save your coziest pajamas (we like Carter's terry onesies with built-in feet) for nighttime only. We swear they induce deep sleep.
- **Bedtime double feed.** Do this one in a very quiet, dimly lit room. After successful burping, place the twins in their crib(s) for bed. Have some dinner, digest, and put yourself to bed (aim for a five-hour chunk).
- **Middle-of-the-night shift.** Since you will probably be out of sorts during this feeding, you can loosen up a bit and feed the twin who's awake first. Enjoy the one-on-one time, put Twin A to sleep, and wake up Twin B for a feeding. After you put Twin B to sleep, close your eyes and dream of getting eight hours.

Staggered

Twin A is fed, changed, and put down to play. Then Twin B is fed, changed, and put down to play while Twin A is put to sleep. Then Twin B is put to sleep.

Pros: *Allows Mom to spend one-on-one time with each twin and really get to know their personalities.*
Cons: Hard to pull off if you don't have an extra helper (Dad, Grandma, or a babysitter) for handing off Twin A. Leaves very little downtime for Mom during the day to attend to other children or responsibilities.

A Staggered Routine

- **Early morning feed.** Start with the twin who wakes up first. It may take a while (around twenty minutes) for you to feed, burp, and change Twin A before you get to Twin B. Put Twin A back down to sleep in crib or bassinet while you are allowing Twin B to wake up naturally by unswaddling. Repeat the routine of feed, burp, change, and back to sleep for Twin B. Then fix yourself a good breakfast and catch a nap if you don't have other kids who will be waking shortly to go to school or morning activities.

- **Late morning feed.** With some luck this will be about three hours from when you started feeding Twin A during the last go-round. Again, feed Twin A first and then Twin B. After they are both fed, give them a sponge bath one at a time with cotton balls on their faces, eyes, ears, and necks. Then take a washcloth to get the other creases on their bodies. Following the sponge bath, put each baby down for a second nap. Repeat with the remaining twin.

- **Lunchtime feed.** Start with Twin A, then finish with Twin B, putting each down for a nap afterward. Ultimately, the hope is that this nap becomes a long one. To encourage the babies to sleep well, swaddle each one and put them in their crib(s). Eat a healthy lunch and then, if you have other kids in school or some sort of backup person watching them, this may be another good chance for you to catch some much-needed sleep.

- **Late afternoon.** When the twins wake up from their nap, feed them separately (starting with Twin A) and enable them to interact on a play mat with some toys after they are burped and changed. All babies have their own fussy times, and this part of the day might be particularly challenging for you. One or both of your twins might resist taking a fourth nap at this time and may stay awake until you feed them again around dinnertime. Even if you're busy soothing two fusspots, remember to drink water and have a power snack.

- **Dinnertime.** After staggered feedings (beginning with Twin A), take the opportunity to give them each a real bath in the baby tub. It may take about an hour to get them both washed, moisturized, massaged, and dressed. Set aside the time to do this every night if you can. This might mean you need to shift your other kids' dinner hour to earlier than they are used to. They can be doing homework, playing computer games, or relaxing while you are rubbing the twins down lovingly. When you are ready to put the twins to sleep, swaddle them again with the hope that this time will ultimately become their permanent bedtime as older babies (meaning that they will eventually sleep for an eight-, ten-, or twelve-hour stretch). Sit down, eat dinner, and drink some water.

- **Mom's bedtime.** After your twins wake up again from their dinner-hour nap, you can feed them individually, starting with Twin A. This is a quiet, no-talking feed. Swaddling and cribs are recommended, too. After they are both down for the count, Mom can shower and hit the sheets (aim for a five-hour chunk of sleep).

- **Middle of the night.** Since you will probably be exhausted during this feeding, you can loosen up a bit about which twin gets fed first. If Twin B is awake first, by all means go ahead and feed him first, change him, and put him back to sleep. Then wake up Twin A and feed her. Be patient: this feeding may take longer because of your exhaustion and their fussiness. Do what you can beforehand to make it easier on yourself, such as having all of your supplies ready and close by.

SLEEP, INTERRUPTED

Even after you've gotten both twins to sleep through the night, one or both may wake up due to teething, growth spurts, dirty diapers, or illness. Even toddler and preschooler twins can start waking at night if they are potty-training and have to pee, if they've had a bad dream, or if they've fallen out of bed. No matter how

Mommy Doc: What Pediatricians Say About Sleep

Safety About one of every thousand singleton babies succumbs to sudden infant death syndrome (SIDS). Most SIDS deaths occur in infants between two and four months. Studies say that an infant born as a twin has more than twice the risk of SIDS than a singleton, due to the higher incidence of prematurity and low birth weight amongst twins. And there may be a slightly increased risk of a surviving twin dying of SIDS if his or her twin dies of the syndrome.

There's a lot more research to be done on SIDS causes, both environmental and genetic. But experts at the American Academy of Pediatrics recommend steps you can take to reduce your twins' risk at home. Here's what's known to keep SIDS at bay:

- Sleep your babies on their backs in their cribs (not your bed).
- Keep your home relatively cool (around 68–70 degrees in the winter).
- Let babies sleep with pacifiers.
- Don't let babies sleep in the crib with a sleep positioner or a hat on.
- Swaddling is okay until babies start to kick off the blankets, but don't overbundle your babies or let them sleep with a top blanket or comforter.
- Don't let anyone smoke where your babies will be.

For reflux (spitting up), Mommy Doc recommends putting something hard, such as books under the legs of one end of the crib or bassinet to help elevate the baby's head. Then she says you can make a "sling" with a rolled-up blanket that's tucked in on both sides of the crib and covering the baby's legs, so the baby doesn't slide to the bottom of the crib. In addition, she stresses the importance of a firm crib mattress and well-fitting crib sheets.

When babies are no longer swaddled, some parents still want to use a blanket. In this case, Mommy Doc suggests tucking all four corners of the blanket into both sides of the crib and putting the blanket under the baby's arms no higher than her chest. Resist the urge to decorate the crib with stuffed animals and pillows. And if you are going to use bumpers, she says, they should be firm, not pillowy. She recommends looking into the mesh bumpers called Crib Shields made by Breathable Baby. Finally, encouraging tummy time during awake time will help babies develop better muscle control that will help them roll from front to back, and back to front in their cribs. Around six months, most babies will be strong enough to position themselves in their cribs however they choose.

old your twins are, it's no fun for you to get a broken night's sleep. Here are some quick fixes for surviving the night and getting through the next day. Adjust to your twins' ages and stages, as needed.

Things to Try if Only One Twin Is Awake

Do the scoop-and-run. Take the crying twin out of the crib or room and bring him into another room to perform triage (dispense Motrin, apply teething gel, change diaper or PJs, give a sip of water). If you bring him into your room, Dad can help by soothing your crying baby while you scramble for remedies.

Decide where baby will sleep for the remainder of the night. That twin can sleep at the foot of your bed in a portable crib or back in the twins' room. This last option is risky: your baby may wake up her twin.

Things to Try if They're Both Awake

Divide and conquer. Wake up your partner and have him hold and comfort one baby in one room while you do the same for the other in a different room. Keep them separate when you perform triage because twins will sometimes exaggerate their discomfort and cry in competition for a parent's compassion. You may end up shouting directions at your husband down the hallway, like "Check the top shelf of the medicine closet!" which is fine if you're all up anyway but not fine if you have other kids who are still sleeping.

Decide where they will sleep for the rest of the night. You may be best off trying to put them both back in their room. Repeat some steps of your bedtime routine to help them assimilate. Or put Twin A back in the room, wait for her to fall asleep, and then put Twin B back in the room. Another option is having them both sleep in bed with you, but many moms caution against establishing that as a permanent routine.

WHEN TWINS HAVE DIFFERENT NAP NEEDS

For many moms, the twins' nap time is the only rest for the weary in a long day of multiple-child care. It can be stressful when one of them is ready to give up a nap (she just plays in the crib and tries to get her twin's attention), rocking the routine. Babies typically go from three naps down to two by six months of age, two naps down to one by fifteen months, and one to none around thirty months. Naturally, since you are dealing with two little people with their own personalities and physiologies, their nap needs will diverge occasionally—even if they are on a good routine. Below are solutions for napping problems.

Recovery Advice for the Next Day

When you and your twins are accustomed to sleeping through the night, all of you can feel out of whack the day after a night of interruptions. Check out these pointers for getting the gang closer to the regular groove:

- Let the twins sleep as long as possible in the morning, even if that means their first meal is not together or that you will be late to get them to their morning activity (if you have other kids to shuttle, this may not be an option).
- Consider keeping them home from their morning activity or school if you feel they're likely to melt down too easily.
- Try to get the routine back in place by lunchtime. This is critical: you don't want their afternoon nap or snack to be too late because that will affect the bedtime routine. Trust us, if you were up last night, you will want your little darlings snoozing as close to their regular bedtime as possible.
- Give yourself a break during the day. Throw some of your parenting rules out the window if you have to: placate cranksters with bottles, pacifiers, or treats, or give your family the same leftovers for lunch and dinner. Line up some help, too: call in a play date or car pool favor, see if you can hire a last-minute mother's helper to drop by for a couple of hours.

Forced Synchronization

How-to with baby twins. To coerce Twin A to give up a nap to keep pace with Twin B, you can gradually shorten Twin A's nap by fifteen minutes every few days. Plan on giving Twin A some extra TLC until she gets the hang of her new routine. Both twins should be in sync within a couple of weeks. Just avoid putting them in the car or stroller during their old nap time, as that will surely lull Twin A to sleep.

How-to with toddler or preschooler twins. If Twin B is ready to wean off naps entirely, you can replace that last nap with quiet time for both twins. This means Twin A and Twin B

Terrific Twinsight: "Getting our triplets to nap si-
multaneously was our biggest parenting success. It was amazing the first
time all three napped at the same time. And it happened purely because
they all cried and I couldn't console them all at once. I put them in their cribs
and walked out of the room. Within five minutes, they were asleep. I woke
my husband to peek in on them, and we celebrated with a high-five and a
hug outside their room."

are sitting or lying down on the couch or floor and physically
resting while watching TV, listening to soft music, or looking at
books. You may need to sit down with both twins to make sure
that quiet time is actually quiet until they get used to it. Even if
they cooperate with quiet time, the dinner hour may become
temporarily challenging because they are tired. Give yourself
an advantage by doing the dinner prep work earlier in the day
and getting the meal on the table a little earlier than your old
routine called for. Bath time and bedtime may end up being a bit
earlier, too.

Making Space for Different Routines

How-to with baby twins. When Twin B wants to play and
Twin A wants to sleep, you can keep them both in their cribs
so long as Twin B doesn't disrupt Twin A's sleep. If Twin B is
disruptive, you can relocate him to a play yard in another bedroom for some quiet playtime or keep him close by so you can
have some one-on-one time. Twin B may be ready to take his
next nap a little earlier than Twin A, so put Twin B down and
spend some special time with Twin A until she is ready for another

rest. Twin A will eventually drop a nap and catch up with Twin B's routine.

How-to with toddler or preschooler twins. Twin A can still take that last nap if Twin B cooperates with your quiet-time rules and doesn't drive you crazy or disturb Twin A. Ideally, Twin B will enjoy having quiet time without Twin A, and you can still manage to decompress or get a few things accomplished. Twin B may be crankier during the dinner hour, so you may want to make it earlier than your old routine called for. If you make Twin A's afternoon snack a little lighter, she may be more open to eating dinner earlier with Twin B. Plan on putting Twin B to bed first and then Twin A.

WHEN TWINS TRANSITION FROM CRIBS TO BEDS

Cribs provide twins with safety and their moms with sanity. So when a mom's daily MO is all about keeping her twins safe, it's tough to let go of the refuge a crib offers and to deal with the freedom a bed allows. In fact, 40 percent of our survey respondents said they found the transition to beds harder for them than they thought it must be for parents of singletons, due at least in part to the fact that twins egg each other on in exploring their newfound freedom. It's easy to slip out and run, it's hilarious to sit up and see your partner in crime touching her toes across the way, and it's fun to jump on your bed—or, even better, from yours to your twin's. In discussing bedtime, one mom from our survey said, "I had no problems until they were about two, and then they really started to work each other up and get into trouble together." Even if just one of your twins is ready to make the change from crib to bed, consider transitioning them together because the one left behind will find it much easier to climb out when he has an enabler at the ready. Eighty-eight percent of our survey respondents agreed that it's best to transition both twins together.

Christina's twins were eighteen months when they turned crib evacuation into an Olympic sport. Although Christina's solution was to put her twins in toddler beds, she has plenty of friends with twins who urged her to consider crib tents instead. (Crib tents are made of mesh netting supported by a frame that attaches to the top of a crib. The tent is opened and closed with a zipper. Check out onestepahead.com or leapsandbounds.com.) They thought Christina's twins were too young to handle the freedom that toddler beds provide. And they were right. The first six months of having her twins in toddler beds was a nightmare—perhaps the lowest point of her twin parenting experience. She dreaded naptime and bedtime because it sometimes took over an hour to get them to settle down and sleep. Christina still wishes she'd tried the tents, thinking that they would have kept her twins in cribs until they were more mature and ready to handle beds better.

Thrival Tip: If your twins stop napping entirely, the moms we surveyed suggest you figure out how you will get a regular break from the twins. This could mean a few hours of preschool each week, a drop-off gymnastics class once a week, and/or a standing play date with a neighbor (one week at your home, one week at hers).

You might consider crib tents if you find yourself in a twin parenting situation that compromises your family's sleep. As one mom said, "Without crib tents, when my triplets were twenty-two months to thirty-six months, they were in danger of either falling out of the cribs or having their mother get so frustrated with their nighttime antics." Similarly, another mom adds, "One had fallen out, which caused injury. Tents were our only option. Though I wrestled with the idea that they were in cages." Seventeen percent of the moms we surveyed said they used crib tents to keep their toddler twins in cribs just a little longer and help ease the transition to beds by moving slightly more mature twins.

HOW TO GET YOUR TWINS TO *STAY* IN BED

Despite spending virtually all waking hours together, many twins have a really hard time calming down at the end of the day; it's just too tempting to slip right out of bed and play with their best buddy in the next bed. If bedtime is becoming a slumber party, without the slumber part, consider these strategies.

Find a bed arrangement that works. That could mean:

- **As far across the room as possible.** Twins may not be able to see each other this way, which may backfire and inspire cross-room consulting to see what the other is up to. On the upside, this will keep twins from jumping bed to bed.
- **Side by side with a bit of space for you to monitor in the middle (Christina's choice).** You can stand in between the beds and rub backs, sing songs, and quietly monitor behavior until both are asleep. However, this may undo all the hard work you put in to get them to self-soothe as babies.
- **Two beds pushed together or one big bed.** This eliminates across-the-room curiosity and fosters physical proximity that some

Eureka! That's Genius! Two Practical Solutions to Twin Toddler Sleep Problems

When Cathy's twins were sixteen months they thought it was a riot to rock their cribs so hard that they'd actually move across the wooden floor. This dynamic duo then tried to reach things on top of the dresser or the air conditioner in the window. To keep the boys' cribs stationary and safe, Cathy's husband bought eight rubber squares, one for each leg of the cribs ($1 for a package of four at Home Depot). Although they are meant to keep furniture from marking a rug, they worked well at curtailing the behavior her guys were trying to get away with.

One mom from our survey said that when her twins were in their twos, they started causing lots of trouble in their cribs. "They became creative with their diapers and throwing things at each other. I put their PJs on backward so they couldn't take off their diapers and have diaper fights." Our financial expert (whom you'll meet in our "Money" chapter, page 242), says he routinely dressed his sons in backward pajamas *and* backward diapers because they were so good at removing their outerwear.

twins still need at night. A possible downside is that this could turn into a big trampoline.

- **Mattresses right on the floor.** It may feel unconventional to you, but they may love the camping-out feel. And you won't have to worry they'll get hurt falling out of bed due to the antics, so particularly at the outset, this may be a great way to make the transition to big-kid beds.

Find the best strategy for putting the twins to bed. Here are some examples:

- **Tucking them in together.** At the end of the day, this can create a very warm and loving group dynamic. If they are not together, some twins always wonder where the other is. Once they are both asleep, you are golden. A joint routine could include dinner, bath, pajamas, quiet playtime, teeth brushing, going to the potty, and story time together.
- **Individual time with each twin.** Even if you are going to put them to bed separately, you can try to get them ready for bed together (baths, teeth brushing, and potty) to save time. If you are the only adult on bedtime duty, set one twin up in a room with a baby monitor with a quiet activity, such as puzzles, coloring, or reading, and read to the other in her bed. This could be your most special one-on-one time of the entire day. If Daddy's home for tuck-ins, you can read to one and he can read to the other. You can give both twins a good-night kiss.

Set some ground rules. If you're consistent in how you put your twins to bed, they'll know what's expected of them when it's time to shut down for a nap or the night, regardless of how tired or rowdy they are. For refusing to go to or stay in bed, enforce

How Long Should Bedtime Take?

Some nights at Christina's home, twin tuck-in takes ten minutes, and other nights it takes up to an hour. There are lots of variables, even if she sticks to their daily routine, including how physically active they were that day, if one or both took a quick car nap, and if their older sister keeps barging in to interrupt with questions like "Are they asleep yet?" What she has noticed is that on nights when they are overtired and up too late, it takes longer to get them to calm down and sleep. Our moms shared how long it usually takes to get both twins down for the count in their homes: up to ten minutes, 37 percent; between ten and twenty minutes, 25 percent; between twenty and thirty minutes, 24 percent; and thirty minutes or more, 16 percent.

consequences like losing certain privileges (no good-night round of Candy Land, or no sweets the next day).

Experiment with policing strategies. Here are a few that may work for you.

- **Stay in the room for a little while.** You can be as unobtrusive as sitting in the corner or as involved as going from bed to bed rubbing tummies or singing lullabies.
- **Leave the room and allow them free rein to get it out of their systems.** This may be more appealing than continually putting twins back in bed and getting frustrated that they're not listening. The first few nights might require parental visits to tuck them in again, but after a while the twins should get over the novelty and fall asleep. One mom told us she literally nailed the furniture to the walls so there would be no safety hazards, then allowed them the freedom to fall asleep at their own pace. The upside: almost every night they'd end up cozied together in her daughter's bed.

Twincidentals: Giving Boy/Girl Twins Their Own

Rooms One mom who answered our survey separated her boy/girl twins very early on because one twin simply didn't sleep as well as the other. Our Mommy Doc separated her boy/girl twins when her other two kids were old enough to want in on the "sleep-over party," which meant that none of them was getting any sleep. If you are a parent of boy/girl twins, Daddy Doc suggests following their cues regarding privacy. "Most boy/girl twins ask for separate rooms by kindergarten," he says. "At that point, they begin to have more different lives: different friends, different activities, and different interests." How can you make the transition easier on twins? You can remind them that separate bedrooms are an upgrade, not a punishment. You can let them have a big say in their new decor and bedding. And, as many moms of older boy/girl twins have told us, make sure at least one twin has room for the other to sleep over whenever they want. A final note from Mommy Doc is to think about timing. "I would not separate twins right before kindergarten starts if they are going to be in separate classrooms. It's too many changes at once," she says.

7

CLEAN KIDS

two children sure generate a lot of mess. Lest your life become an endless battle against food-covered faces, dirty clothes, and used sippy cups, we offer from-the-trenches advice to help you prepare for, handle, and minimize the chores. A good starting point is cleaning your two little mess makers themselves.

KEEPING TWIN BODIES BRIGHT AND SHINY

Take two babies and add water and before you know it, you have a slip-'n'-slide adventure. Between the squirminess and the slipperiness, your babies can feel like a couple of eels. Water always demands parents' full attention, but parents of twins also need to factor in logistical challenges: Where is the other baby while you are bathing his or her twin? And how do you safely get one out at a time when they are sharing the tub?

Feedback from the moms we've surveyed has been mixed. Many say bathing twins is nerve-racking, one of the most stressful things a parent can do; others say it's no big deal and even go so far as to describe the process as relaxing. Chances are you'll find yourself moving from one end of the spectrum to the other on a daily basis.

Different ages and stages demand different strategies: newborns may be easiest to bathe one at a time, yet both you and your toddlers may prefer the group dynamic. For many moms, bathing the twins at night provides a great way to reconnect after the sometimes arduous chore of the dinner hour. Others prefer the morning because of the fresh start it can offer after a tough night of sleep (or lack thereof).

Our preferred method for tub time involves a helper (Dad, older sibling, babysitter, Grandma, etc.) who can whisk a wet baby in his or her towel to the changing station for a clean diaper, warm PJs, and loving kisses. But that is not always an option; a full 44 percent of the moms we surveyed said they always give babies their baths with no extra help. To maximize bath time bonding and your focus on the twins' safety, consider these general bathing tips.

- **Implement an out-of-the-box bath schedule.** Especially for moms bathing the babies on their own, rotating bath nights, one baby every other night, can really make things more manageable. Other moms report that bathing babies when you have time during the day makes a huge difference. Morning baths can be a nice fresh start to each day, and older siblings are more likely to be out of the house at school or activities. Try bathing babies in the middle of the day, after lunch and before the long afternoon nap. Or consider a flexible routine that takes advantage of help whenever it's available.
- **Use a combination bath wash instead of body soap and shampoo,** such as Johnson's Head-to-Toe (a survey favorite). You already have two babies to wash; why follow a two-step process, too?

- **Pare down your bath toys** to avoid being overwhelmed by children and rubber duckies.
- **Make sure you have all your supplies within arm's reach** before bringing your babies into the water, including the post-bath towels and diapers.
- **Consider installing a removable handheld sprayer** in the sink or tub to make rinsing easier. If that is not an option, keep a small cup or bowl nearby.
- **Give sponge baths as an alternative to the tub,** even when your twins are older, on the evenings when you are limited to one set of hands, or if you just need a break from the regular routine.
- **Take advantage of the great outdoors.** During the summer, an outdoor hose-down or shower (look at Home Depot, Costco, or a Frontgate catalogue for an outdoor shower you can install yourself) can be a great way to rinse the day away. Christina's twins, as babies, loved a summer bath in their plastic turtle pool on the patio.

AGE-SPECIFIC BATH BASICS

Cleaning Newborns and Infants

Incorporate sponge baths and washcloth rubdowns. Moms want to keep babies' navel areas clean and dry when they first come home from the hospital, but even after the cords fall off and it's safe to give your babes regular baths, sponge baths and/or washing with a cloth can still be the way to go. They're easier for you, many babies seem less averse to the warm cloth than to the tub, and they can be done right on the changing table surface, utilizing a small bowl of warm water.

Cathy's baby nurse taught her to incorporate daily sponge baths into the midday routine, which signaled to her boys that nap time was on its way. She would strip each boy to his diaper, make sure the washcloth was soaked in warm water, and lift all their little appendages to get into the crevices. Afterward, she would help the boys transition into nap mode by applying calming lotion or giving a short massage to each baby.

Bathe babies one at a time until they are big and strong enough to sit up on their own. This begs the question of how you keep the other twin occupied and happy when you are bathing one twin. We both set up our twins together in one crib while we prepared for bath time. While waiting for the bathing process to begin, our twins would interact with each other or watch an overhead mobile in the crib. We stripped them down to their diapers, left them in the crib until the tub and all necessary equipment were completely ready, and then gave one bath at a time. Sometimes the one left behind would cry, and those were the nights we practiced speed bathing and postponed our individual bonding time until the nighttime feeding or tuck-in.

Select the right location. Needless to say, bathing can pose some logistical challenges with twins. Here are some places to try that are both safe and practical:

- **In the shower with you.** Many of the moms we surveyed said they found peace cleaning their babies in the shower. You can leave one child safely tucked in a baby seat, swing, or crib, or later in an activity center such as the ExerSaucer, and then wash one baby with you at a time. One mom told us she keeps the waiting twin in the laundry basket right next to the tub; another pulls a high chair right into the bathroom so the waiting twin is sitting up, watching the fun. Dry the baby and hand her off to your waiting partner or place her safely on a thick blanket or bath mat, then go for round two. The advantages of this method include great one-on-one bonding as you cradle your baby in your arms and the fact that three family members get clean with one run of the water. The downside is that babies are *very* slippery when wet and soapy, so be careful!

- **In infant tubs.** Finally, something you can get away with buying only one of! Like many of the moms we surveyed, Cathy bathed one twin at a time using an infant tub in the bathroom sink until the babies were big enough to tip the tub over (around three months). You can also place the infant tub in your regular tub instead of the sink, but be careful because that can be tough on your back. Some moms even put an infant tub in the shower with them. Look for the infant tubs that have hammocks or slings or pillows to help keep slippery newborn bodies propped up and in place; it makes it easier for you to wash them safely.

- **In the kitchen sink.** Deep sinks, especially those with side-by-side sections, are perfect for little bodies. Use a handheld sprayer for a gentle rinse. The kitchen sink is also a good option if you have other children who can play or watch TV within earshot (if not eyeshot) to minimize distractions during bath time. This is a very popular choice, and it's what Christina did when her babes were small. Buy a waterproof pillow or roll up a towel to cushion and support your babies' heads. You'll still need to do alternating twin baths, but it is nice to be able to keep the non-bather nearby and in a comfortable space (such as in the swing in the kitchen or an adjoining family room). This is where multiple changing stations really help, too. Create your own space on the floor or set up a changing station near the kitchen and stock it with PJs and other needed items.

Use bath seats. As your babies grow, so do your bathing options. Babies who can sit up confidently but who are not yet ready to control themselves on the tub floor are ideal candidates for seats or rings (a favorite of our respondents). Cathy used two plastic ring seats by Safety 1st. Several of the moms we surveyed favor the softer seats made by Leachco. You can fit two rings in your regular family tub at the same time, so your babies can finally look each other in the eye and splash together. This is when bath time transitions from endearing one-on-one time for you and each twin to fun time for the twins with each other. But with two seats in the tub, it is close quarters, so one baby is probably going to end up somewhere near the tub spout. Many of the moms we surveyed solved this problem with a soft spout cover so their babies' heads are protected.

This is a great stage for parents, too, because they can finally save some time and merge two baths into one. With two babies in the tub, however, someone has to be removed first, which means someone is left behind in the tub. If you have the seats properly secured to the tub and the babies properly secured in the seats, you can drain the bath and dry off and diaper one twin near the tub while the other waits in the tub. But be careful once they learn to shimmy the seat to a spot near the faucet—some babies find hot water handles fascinating. Plus, active babies can tip the rings over, especially when there is no water in the tub, so take caution.

A downside of rings and seats is that your twins' little tushies never seem to get as clean as they do when just soaked in a tub without a seat. And the seats certainly take up space if you need the tub and bathroom to function for people besides your twins.

Blow up an inflatable tub. Several of the moms we surveyed utilized tubs and pools. Leachco makes the Bath 'N Bumper inflatable tub (a favorite), as well as a variety of other inflatable bath products. The inflatable tub fits right inside your standard tub and is made for one baby to use at a time after outgrowing the infant tub. One advantage of inflatable tubs and pools is that they can be deflated and hung to dry, taking up much less space than plastic seats and tubs.

Rub-a-Dub-Dub, Twin Toddlers in the Family Tub

Once your twins are mature enough to sit together in the tub while you bathe them, the real fun begins. You can sing songs, play with bubbles, and let them wash each other's hair (although that sometimes ends badly) and enjoy each other's company. On the flipside, we feel we've exhausted every possible method for avoiding getting soaked, to no avail. Just as two toddlers sleeping in the same room technically constitute a slumber party, two toddlers in the same tub could easily be mistaken for a pool party. They are naked and unconstrained—what could be better? Throw in a few bath toys, and from their perspective you are basically asking for trouble, right? Do not bathe your twins in an outfit you intend to wear past bath time.

Take twins out one at a time. Even if your twins can walk and stand unassisted, you should drain the water and guide them out of the tub one at a time. Handing one child off to Dad or a

Thrival Tip: Sliding glass shower doors can seriously limit your reach into the bathtub since the ideal washing spot is right in the center of the tub, between your twins. One mom told us she and her husband removed the sliding doors for better bathing. It might seem extreme, but it's temporary and will probably end up saving your back and the doors in the long run.

babysitter is an ideal solution, but if you're bathing your twins alone, you'll need to figure out how to balance getting one safely out while still keeping a hand and eye on the one still in the tub. Try setting up two different color bath mats or towels on the floor. Ask the first child out of the tub to stand on her assigned spot. Wrap her in a towel that has a hood so there's a chance of it staying in place.

Beware of clean twins on the loose. Once they are out of the tub, the routine you might have developed (drying them off and diapering them right in the bathroom) starts to blow some leaks. Twins who *can* walk *want* to walk. There is no sound as heart-stopping as the sound of your toddler's head hitting the tile floor after a nasty slip with wet feet in a wet bathroom. To prevent accidents, you can keep the bathroom door closed, so there's nowhere for an antsy twin to escape, keep toys by the assigned bath mat to keep the antsy twin busy, and spread extra towels on the floor to provide water absorption and an extra cushion in case of a wipeout. (For more about accident prevention, see our "Safety Matters" chapter on page 231.)

Bathe all your kids together. When Cathy's twins were around eighteen months, it became feasible to bathe all four of her boys together. Yes, it is tight, and the older boys need to be especially careful of the twins, but it is so much fun. They love it, especially with bubbles. It's nice to have the younger guys bond with the older guys. She doesn't do it every night, but it makes for some great family photos in this setting.

Three Reasons to Evacuate the Tub—Fast!

1. **Meltdowns.** When a mother is bathing a singleton child and he or she goes into meltdown mode, it's challenging to quickly get him or her out of the tub. For parents of twins, it's virtually impossible: someone is always left behind in the slippery tub. Sometimes allowing the upset child to stand up and give you a hug is the remedy you need; other times it means emptying the tub fast. At least quickly rinsed babies are better than dirty ones.

2. **Poop in the tub.** Just like at the public pool, this means everyone out of the water. Hose or wipe them down to rinse off the dirty water, dry and dress them, and put them in a safe place before you disinfect the scene of the crime. Try again tomorrow.

3. **Fighting.** Between preferred seating and bath toys, moms can end up spending more time refereeing than cleaning their twins. Sometimes pulling the plug on the bath is the only way to put the kibosh on a twin tub brawl, especially if they are tired at the end of a long day.

"THE LAUNDRY HAS MADE ME CRY"

That is a direct quote from one of the mothers we surveyed. Before the twins, maybe you were used to just yourself and your partner generating dirty clothes, with one or two laundry days per week. Then the twins are born and you're a family of four, with more than twice the laundry you had before. Day in and day out, that's a minimum of two onesies, two outfits, two sweaters, four socks, etc. All of a sudden, you have one day a week that is assigned for *not* doing laundry! The best advice our moms give: it's better to plow through the laundry than dig out from under it. Read on for tips to deal with this most tedious of chores.

Don't skip a day. Okay, maybe we're exaggerating a little, but not much. The best method of managing the laundry is keeping it in constant forward motion. Between you, your partner, and your two children (at a minimum), you'll be generating a justifiable load of dirty clothes just about every day.

Mix it up. One mom told us she opts not to dress her twin girls in matching outfits because it helps clothes go further, a laundry- and money-saving tip. Coordinating outfits require planning and is yet another restriction on your ability to be flexible, but they do look adorable. We suggest saving the coordinated outfits for special occasions or days when you want some familial twin attention.

Don't let fear of laundry tempt you into buying more clothes. There are days when the twins go through several outfit changes each, but many other days when one outfit makes it through a whole day. One mom told us she changed her infants' clothes only when they were actually dirty, which for some babies means an outfit could last more than a day. As long as your laundry is moving forward, chances are you have enough pairs of pants yourself every morning, too. Worst-case scenario: you all wear something two days in a row.

Find a place for clean clothes. Many moms tell us they have little trouble getting the clothes in and out of the washer and dryer; it's the folding and putting away of clean clothes that trips them up. Consider keeping a clean laundry basket where clothes come out of the dryer and wait to go right onto the body of a twin. Cathy piles her clean clothes on top of her bed so she can't climb in until the clothes are put away. It may seem like a sick kind of self-punishment, but it works for her.

Thrival Tip: Avoid the task of matching multiple pairs of clean baby socks by buying one type for each twin. You can assign by color or brand so there's no folding and no confusion.

CLEANING UP SPILLS AND THRILLS AT HOME

Once we had children, our homes became a little messier than we had ever anticipated—with toys strewn across the floors, beds unmade, and piles of laundry waiting to be folded—but at least things were always more or less clean and sanitary underneath the mess. Our twins, especially as toddlers, have moved us right into downright dirty. It's not easy to keep up with the spilled drinks and mashed-up crackers while chasing the adorable little slobs around the house.

Cathy loves when her mom comes to visit because her mom can't stand the sight of a messy playroom and will organize and clean. But there is always a high cringe factor when she discovers an old bagel or smelly cup of milk under the pile of Legos and blocks. Cathy rationalizes that "Who raised you?" look in her mother's eyes by reminding herself that even though her mother had four kids, she never had twins.

Here's some advice for cleaning up your especially dirty situations.

Adopt a strategy of containment. One of the most challenging things to deal with is toddler twin cyclones trailing you as you attempt to clean and organize your home. You make the beds in one room, they pull clothes out of the closet in another; you go to pick up the clothes and put them back in the closet, they spill water on the beds you just made.

You can curtail this mess-making merriment by containing your twins in a playpen or distracting them with a favorite game or toy when you are trying to clean up. Limit their toys to one or two rooms and designated storage bins or boxes. Attempt to limit food to a few rooms, such as the kitchen and family room. Same goes for where you decide to store things that they like to pull out: if you can deal with cleaning up Tupperware over and over again, leave that in the low cabinets. If you can't keep them away from the unopened rolls of toilet paper, move them up higher (see our "Safety Matters" chapter on page 231 for more twin-proofing tips). And definitely invest in some childproofing equipment. Don't worry, the plastic locks on your cabinets are temporary (twins seem to be most curious between the ages of twelve months and three years).

Keep the situation in perspective. Remember, you are dealing with twice the spilled milk, twice the thrown spaghetti, and twice the crayon experiments gone bad. Staying on offense instead of always playing defense is the right mind-set, but cut yourself some slack if you find yourself behind the curve every few days. Just keep doing laundry. (We're only half kidding.)

MEALTIME MESSES

Do the math: two babies, three meals each, and maybe one or two snacks a day. That's somewhere between six and twelve cleanups daily! Cleaning up food (whether left over, dropped, thrown, or spit out) is one of the least appealing things about parenthood. And you get to do it all twice as often as the average parent. Sometimes we feel like all we do is clean up after messy meals. Days later, we can still find dried pasta or smeared applesauce on the walls. Somehow it seems as if the chairs themselves ingest as much food as the babies. The straps are impossible to keep clean. That having been said, we recommend that you try to clean the chairs after every meal because, like laundry, skipping a few cleanups can snowball and one day it all catches up with you when you realize your babies are sitting in garbage. But there are some things you can do to make cleanups easier down the road.

Consider wooden high chairs. When her twins were twelve months, Christina got fed up with her hard-to-clean high chairs and went old-school. She bought two Kettler chairs and decided to go cushionless. Wooden chairs are easier to keep clean than the bulky plastic ones with vinyl-covered cushions, and most slide in nicely to a standard table so your twins can really enjoy family dining with the rest of you. But the chairs that Christina bought only had simple lap belts that could not prevent her son from climbing out when he was eighteen months. Her son frequently escaped (sometimes covered in food), and her daughter cheered him on from her chair. Be a smart shopper: Eddie Bauer and Safety 1st make wooden chairs with three-point harnesses that might better restrain toddlers.

Look for tray inserts. Cathy bought her twins the Peg Perego Prima Pappas, plastic chairs with tray inserts that fit on the removable top. The trays are easy to remove and clean. The Eddie Bauer wooden model also offers a removable insert.

Keep the chairs in the same feeding zone at all times. It's great that some high chairs have wheels for easy maneuverability, but since your twins will make messes while they are eating, we recommend minimizing the square footage of your mess. The floor under our twins' chairs is pretty gross, but at least it's not the whole room. To avoid permanent stains on the carpet or sticky

Five Ways to Minimize Twin Meal Messes

1. Keep a supply of baby wipes near the high chairs.
2. Use plastic bibs with pockets to catch stray crumbs.
3. Keep your twins eating in high chairs as long as you can.
4. Invest in both a handheld vacuum and a broom/picker-upper.
5. Don't free them from the seats until you've cleaned the trays and the floor around them.

floors, some moms like using easy-clean plastic mats under the twins' chairs.

Think outside the chair. One mom suggests a plastic picnic table in the kitchen instead of high chairs as an option for toddler twins. The table is easier to clean and doubles as an art and activity center.

KEEPING YOUR CAR CLEAN (SORT OF)

Try to rule your ride. Sticking to your guns about no eating in the car is a little bit easier to do when you're exerting control over one screaming toddler. But two screaming toddlers can drive you to cave on your own rules. Just remember: enforcing rules, when you have the patience, does help cut down on the mess.

Take advantage of opportunities for damage control. Between stray mittens and toys, crumbs, dirty snow or sand, and a trunk jammed with sports equipment, clothes to be donated, and a double stroller, our cars can get really gross. It helps to keep a car vacuum fully charged. And many car wash places offer discounts if you go during off-peak times, such as during dinner hours. Or buy a multipack of washes at a reduced rate.

Safer Cleaners

Babies require a lot of equipment for both transport and entertainment. Car seats, swing seats, ExerSaucers, and Jumperoos are all full of nooks, crannies, and much-harder-to-remove-than-advertised removable covers perfect for catching spit-up and food. After a while, they can smell bad and get crusty. Using very hot water and clear dish soap works and is safe in case babies chew or suck on parts of these items. Running removable pieces through the dishwasher or washing machine can also help. Another motivational tool for cleaning purposes: twins can pass germs back and forth frequently.

White vinegar is a great way to clean heavy-duty messes. It disinfects and deodorizes and is safe and cheap. You can use it on carpets and other fabrics straight from the bottle or mix it with water for a cleaning solution safe for ExerSaucers and plastic toys. It can even be run through your clothes washer to keep it fresh after heavy use. When Christina's twins had rotavirus (which created severe tummy trauma from both ends for a week), she went through at least a gallon of white vinegar. You can also check out your local grocery store for natural cleaning products that can safely handle the dirtiest jobs.

Put junk in its place. People have remarked to Cathy that her car is remarkably clean for someone who has four boys, which probably means it's only slightly messy. One way she manages the wrappers, straws, and tissues in the car is to keep a small trash bag in the front seat. Some moms go so far as to implement mini storage systems in their trunks for toys or boots or cleaning supplies.

8

PEE AND POOP

Of the many unglamorous aspects of motherhood, constantly wiping twin butts ranks pretty high on the list. While you may not find changing diapers or toilet training too personally rewarding, it's part of the job, and with twins, there are times when even this mundane task can turn into a bit of a circus act. Our advice is to make the best of it: try to enjoy the one-on-one time when you're diapering one baby and the bonding time when you find yourself locked in the bathroom with one or more toddlers who are learning to use the toilet. Read on to find out how you can make the job a little more efficient, if not glamorous.

DIAPERING INFANTS AND NEWBORNS

We were floored by how many diapers we used in a twenty-four-hour period (around twenty a day during the first few weeks), by how much time it took us to change our babies and any soiled clothes or linens, and by how much our backs hurt from bending over all the time. The good news is that the quantity of diapers

Mommy and Daddy Doc: It's important to

stay on top of both the number and details of babies' diapers, especially during the first few weeks home from the hospital, primarily as a marker of hydration and nutrition. Mommy Doc says each twin should have four to eight wet diapers and two to three poops during this crucial time. For newborns, especially breast-fed ones, it can be challenging for parents to be certain how much liquid their infants are getting during each feeding. Daddy Doc adds: "Doctors look at indirect measures of nutrition, and what is coming out in terms of poop and pee becomes a really good way to track how much the infant is getting in. This is very important since twins tend to be smaller at birth, so doctors are very interested in how much weight they are gaining."

definitely decreases as babies get older and start eating solid foods, so backbreaking labor is a temporary situation. Here are lots of tips to help alleviate diapering frustrations.

Minimize the Impact on Your Wallet

Buy in bulk. If you've never belonged to a warehouse club before, now is the time to join. In our survey, moms mention Costco, Sam's Club, and BJ's. You can find diapers, wipes, butt cream, formula, and other baby essentials (even organic baby food) at these wholesale stores, so the accumulated savings over time is certainly worth the initial membership fee. And don't be afraid to load up when you're there; when shopping for baby basics, we typically buy at least twice the amount we need, to save ourselves a shopping trip later. Wipes, in particular, are everywhere—in our homes, cars, and bags. We each have one full backup box from Costco (with 704 wipes) just in case.

Go online. You can buy Pampers and Huggies diapers online wholesale at 1800diapers.com. An extra-large case of Pampers Baby-Dry (198 diapers) sells online for about half the price of drugstore-bought packages. Shipping is free if you spend over $50, and they have a great "refer-a-mom" program.

Utilize coupons. Pampers offers a type of frequent-flyer discount club, the "Gifts to Grow" program, that benefits mothers who purchase a lot of diapers. You collect codes from the packages of diapers you buy, then redeem them online from the Pampers rewards catalog. If you sign up on the Huggies Web site, they'll send you coupons, too. But learn from other moms' most common mistake: the trick with paper coupons is to use 'em or lose 'em (we've lost many). Keep them readily accessible in your wallet or in a purse-size organizer to help you remember to use them before they expire.

Shop smarter. This is a case when you may have to weigh cost against convenience. For example, you might be able to quickly fill prescriptions by running in to your local pharmacy, so it would be easiest to grab a package of diapers when you're there anyway. It might take you more effort (driving time and gas) to get to one of the bigger general retail chains like Target or Wal-Mart, which typically sell large packages of diapers at significantly cheaper prices. But the double diaper bucks add up over the years, so make the effort to find your cheapest spot and stock up. Particularly when your twins are older, and they stay in one-size diapers for an extended period of time, it's really worth it. (Check out our "Money" chapter, page 242, for more ways to save with twins.)

Simplify When You Can

The frequency of babies' peeing and pooping means you spend a lot of time diapering (infants should have six to eight changes each per day), so anything you can do to streamline the process will lighten the load on your psyche.

Create multiple diaper-changing stations. Sixty-three percent of the moms we surveyed said setting up more than one diaper-changing station at home was a top mommy secret. Put stations wherever it makes the most sense for you. It may be that you need one each on the first and second floors of your home to avoid having to carry both twins up and down the stairs. Or you may need one in the play area, or wherever you spend most of your time with babies, and one in your bedroom, where babies are temporarily sleeping.

Try to make sure those stations are always fully stocked with bed linens, diaper changing pads, wipes, diapers, ointment, onesies and other comfy baby clothes, Purell, and bundling blankets. You'll be surprised at how fast your two babies go through your surplus. Christina's hint: buy a package of diapers in the next size, as one or both of the twins will get there soon.

Be more streamlined on the go. All you need is a lightweight diaper bag with at least four diapers, a small package of wipes, a changing pad, and butt cream. One of our moms says she always brings her diaper bag back in the house with her when she's unloading the car or stroller from a journey with the twins. This way she restocks it immediately and it's ready to grab for the next outing.

Have a low-maintenance approach to babies' bedding. Diapers leak, pajamas and mattress covers get soiled. Be prepared for middle-of-the-night changes by stocking up on extra crib sheets (two for each twin should be fine) and sheet savers (another mommy trick revealed in our survey). Cut down on your multiples' laundry and save time changing their cribs by buying

Twincidentals: **Being Green with Twins** Finding con-

venient, accessible, and affordable baby care methods is a survival skill for moms of twins. But all of the stuff we use to care for our multiples can add to our concerns about our family's impact on the environment. Bigger cars, cans of formula, boxes and jars of baby food—sometimes it feels as if we families of multiples are using more than our share. Take heart, you actually might be more green than you think, and you can always do more to be eco-friendly.

- **Stop worrying about those diapers.** The good news is that today's disposable diapers are doing much more with less raw materials. Over the past twenty years, manufacturers like Pampers have reduced packaging weight by 80 percent, in addition to reducing the amount of materials, energy, and water used. As far as cloth diapers go, recent studies have found little or no difference between the environmental impact of cloth and disposable diapers. If you are curious about cloth diapers, check out clothdiaperinfo.com or diapernet.com. Another option is alternative disposable diapers, available at some natural retailers such as Whole Foods. So feel good about whatever choice you make, and remember, the diaper phase will be over before you know it.

- **Make an enduring environmental contribution by raising two eco-sensitive children.** As they grow, they can help you recycle plastic and glass bottles, cans, batteries, and more. You can also bring them grocery shopping with you and teach them about the benefits of locally grown and organic foods. And you can inspire them to do eco-creative things like turning toilet paper tubes into music shakers.

- **Put your dollars where your conscience is.** You can donate to an organization that supports global warming solutions or you can offset your family's carbon footprint by donating at nativeenergy.com.

non-fitted mattress covers (have one backup for each twin) and two fitted crib sheets for each twin. Skip the dust ruffles, even though they are so cute.

Don't Let Diaper Blowouts Ruin Your Day

Sometimes pee and poop escape the confines of your babies' diapers. Lest your white carpet or even dark brown couch become a literal dumping ground, you need to take immediate action when you spot a baby with a leak. Fortunately, double diaper blowouts are a rare occurrence, so you can probably count on putting one baby safely in a crib or high chair while you deal with the other's mess. Clean the messy baby's body first (with a washcloth rub-down or a quick tub), diaper and dress her, and put her in a safe place (maybe to keep her twin company). Then you can toss the soiled car seat cover or couch pillow in the wash or spot-treat the dirtied non-machine-washable item.

LOGISTICS OF CHANGING TWO BABIES

Small Babies

The assembly-line approach to infant diapering is the way to go. If you feed babies at or around the same time, you can burp as needed, play with each a little bit, and then change one by one. You'll quickly figure out who should get changed first (we say go for the messier, stinkier, or crankier one). You'll also have to figure out what to do with the other baby while you're changing his sibling. When our babies were still really tiny and in need of a diaper change, we'd put both twins in one crib, bassinet, or portable crib, and change them right in there.

Once babies start rolling over, typically around four months of age, two in the crib becomes a messier and less appealing option. This is when we started alternating one baby at a time on the changing table (and leaving the other in a safe spot). It's also the time when their needs start to diverge; you find yourself changing less out of habit or routine and more driven by need. Don't feel bad if you're changing one more than the other; by this time you'll have changed so many diapers it will become a test of speed rather than the cute bonding experience it was a few months ago.

Bigger Babies

Once solids were introduced, our twins drank bottles less frequently (yours may be nursing less often) and started a more structured meal plan. It was an interesting shift—they started pooping less often and playing more often. When they were both engaged in a play activity and we smelled a stinker or saw a full diaper, it was a bummer to disrupt the fun and carry both of them away; the fixed diaper-changing stations became more of a hassle than a helper. During this phase, your best bet is a portable changing basket including diapers, wipes, ointment, and a pad. This way, you can get down on the floor and change one twin while the other is close by experimenting with balls and blocks and change the other as needed. Keep two stocked baskets wherever it makes sense in your home (perhaps one upstairs and one downstairs).

The Sisterhood of the Traveling Changing Station

Unfortunately, diaper duty is one job that isn't limited to the confines of your home. No matter if it's a quick walk around the block or a long road trip to Grandma's house, you've got to be able to deal with dirty diapers *anytime, anywhere*. Luckily, we've got troubleshooting tips that will help you avoid the most common changing mishaps on the go. Here's what to do when:

- **They're buckled up tight in your car in your driveway and one of them has a dirty diaper.** You can take both out of the car and back in the house for the change. Or acknowledge that you've crossed borders: out of the house means you're away from home and reliant on a portable changing station. A diaper mat in the back of your car works well, or you can utilize the empty passenger seat in the front of your car or your SUV hatch (weather permitting) to make the change.
- **You're in a parking lot and you realize one has a yucky bottom.** You can go through the Herculean effort of maneuvering both babies out of the car seats, into a stroller, and into an indoor changing facility at the mall, grocery store, or playground. Or use the supplies in your diaper bag (even if it means cold wipes) for an in-car or in-stroller (if it's not an umbrella-style one) change. Stash plastic grocery or newspaper bags in your car diaper kit and use them for containing dirty diapers, wipes, or soiled clothes.
- **You're at the mall with both children strapped in the side-by-side stroller.** As you casually peruse the latest fashions, you notice a strong smell emanating from down below. One or both of your twins has produced something stinky. You can leave your purchases with a salesclerk to avoid schlepping them with you. Assuming you can reach a restroom via elevator instead of escalators or stairs and can squeeze your double stroller through the doorway, you can use a changing station there or head back to your car. Another reason to keep wipes and diapers in your stroller's storage space or your bag.

Most of our moms report toddler pee or poop moments that are so zany, it's hard for them to figure out what to do first to control the chaos. Christina once walked in on her twins in the playroom with onesies on and snapped but diapers ripped off. There were little poop nuggets everywhere—even in the baskets of toys. The twins must have thrown them around the room. They thought it was great fun; she thought it was so disgusting she started to cry. It took her about an hour to clean up, and the room smelled like Lysol for a week, but she can laugh about it now. We hope you can look back on your twins' diaper madness in a few weeks or months and laugh. For now, you've got to survive this phase and keep on thriving. Help is on the way!

Take a preemptive stance against their mischievousness. You kept diaper-changing supplies close by when your twins were babies, but now it's time to hide that potentially dangerous or messy stuff. Our moms resort to hiding their gear in a drawer or cabinet (sometimes a locked one) or to putting it way up high on the top shelf of a closet. It's inconvenient, but better than worrying that your twins will try feeding the butt paste to each other.

So you don't feel like a total ogre, you can indulge their naughtiness a tad. Part of the fun for toddler twins is showing off for each other and feeling like they're getting away with being naughty, so consider occasionally leaving diapers and wipes around for them to mess up. Wipes can be rescued off the floor, balled up, and shoved in a plastic bag and still work just fine. We each keep 704 around, so it's no big deal!

Head off twin toddlers' poopcapades. One common cause of pee and poop messes is when toddlers remove their own full diapers. If your twins do this, you may need to stop dressing

Twincidentals: Pity Parties

Even with new systems in place to deal with your twin toddlers' diaper-related behavior, you may need to dig deep for patience. Some days you may be able to laugh at your toddlers' poopcapades, and other days they may make you want to cry or yell at your twins. This is all normal. If you're really having a bad day, try not to wallow in your misery or take it out on the twins, but share it with someone—your best friend, your mother-in-law, or us (we're always compassionate at twinsetmoms.com). Or you can say a calming mantra or prayer (Christina and many of our survey respondents are all about "This too shall pass"). Definitely figure out how you can avoid being in the frustrating situation again, or focus on tomorrow being a new day.

them in the easy-off, easy-on clothes that made multiple diaper changes less taxing when they were babies. Instead, consider layering twin toddlers' clothes so they have a harder time getting to their diapers: two onesies with snaps on the bottom, pants with a button or zip fly, or tights with bloomers on top. Or take it as a sign that they're ready to begin potty training.

Sometimes in the event of a pee or poop mess in your home, one or both of your toddler twins may decide they are eager to "help" clean up (translation: grab the squirt bottle of stain remover and spray it in their twin's eye), and it's hard to know what to do first. We've broken the cleanup process down for you into four simple steps:

Step 1. Remove twins from the soiled area (the carpet, the floor, the crib) and clean their bodies off.

Step 2. Make sure they are in clean diapers and clothes so they can't rip off their diapers and start more trouble while you are cleaning up.

Step 3. Put the twins in a safe place and give them each something to occupy them (crib with books, high chair with Cheerios).

Step 4. Clean, disinfect, and deodorize the targets.

THE SUPER BOWL: POTTY-TRAINING TWINS

Potty-training twins is a daunting task; many moms dread the challenge months before their twins even show signs of being ready. Because it can require so much parental patience and persistence and time, some moms we surveyed consider potty-training their twins to be their greatest parenting success. On a similar note, 44 percent of the moms of twins we surveyed ranked their

Daddy Doc: When Boy/Girl Twins Get Curious About Their Privates

Sometimes having a twin of a different gender can promote innocent comments or questions that catch parents off guard. Never fear—Daddy Doc has some insights to share: "Toddlers are naturally curious about their bodies, and also those of their siblings. As parents, we should approach that interest in a non-judgmental, non-embarrassed, matter-of-fact manner. We don't want them to be embarrassed about their bodies, but they do need to learn what is socially acceptable and what isn't. Follow the child's lead with body part questions and deal with them as they come up. The less of a deal we make, the better. Kids know when adults are embarrassed or hiding something, and if they sense that, the issue in question becomes suddenly more fun to them."

potty-training experience as harder to accomplish than the experience of the singleton parents they know. Take heart: Christina's twins, who caused all sorts of trouble with their diaper messes when they were toddlers, were remarkably easy to potty-train. Both were day- and night-trained, without great stress, when they were just over two years old. Miracles do happen!

As we know from personal experience with our older, singleton children, a parent's attitude and approach can make a big difference in the speed with which children get the hang of potty training. Daddy Doc recommends that parents of multiples need to take a laid-back approach: "Potty training goes better and easier when parents don't try to force the issue, but instead let kids take the lead. That relaxed approach seems to be especially important for twins." But it's also true that some children just kind of get it. According to experts, fraternal twins tend to develop slightly differently from each other, and girls tend to train sooner and faster than boys. This was true with Christina's boy/girl twins. Her daughter was three months ahead of her son in day and night training.

The moms we surveyed were evenly split: 50 percent potty-trained their twins together, as one unit, and 50 percent potty-trained their twins individually. Take into account the temperaments of your children, readiness signs, your schedule and their schedule, and the pros and cons of staggering your twins before you decide which route to take. Sometimes having a deadline, such as the start of a preschool or camp that has a no-diapers policy, or the beginning of summer with the lure of a big pool with a no-diaper rule, can inspire a mom or twin to start training. Other times, training one child first could make the other eager to shed his diaper, too. Check out our guide to potty-training basics, with a twin twist.

Basic Training

Look for readiness cues. According to Daddy Doc, most girls are potty-trained between ages two and three, and boys on average tend to be six to nine months later. Most children start to say they're ready by showing general interest in all things potty. This means broadcasting that they're peeing in the tub, pulling off their diapers, telling you when they're wet or dirty, wanting to watch you do your business, or flushing out of curiosity. If one or both of your twins show signs, start training whoever is ready—this may mean separately or together. Regardless, most moms feel pretty strongly that once you start the process you have to follow through. Quite simply, you won't have the time or the energy to choreograph a bunch of false starts.

Stock up on the supplies you'll need. This is probably the most fun part of the process, so grab both twins, even if only one is potty-ready, and go shopping. You should be able to get everything you might need at Wal-Mart or Target, including undies, portable potties for home, and/or the car, toilet insert (pick one that they both like, to keep their small tushies from falling down into the bowl), and stuff to bribe/reward them with. Let them pick out a few things by themselves.

Help them get acquainted with the sensation. Some moms like their twins to be naked around the house or in the backyard to help them get the hang of what it feels like when pee or poop is coming. (This au naturel approach can backfire when you are out in public and your son drops his shorts to take a leak because he doesn't understand the difference between public urination and backyard privacy.) Other moms like to put their kids on the potty or the bowl every hour or so. To make this easier, some moms will put potties in the playroom or in front of the television. Whether you go commando or are bowl-bound, the twins are going to be homebound for a while. You'll know you've hit a major training milestone when they start telling you that they have to go pee or poop, and they actually make it to the potty on time and make pee or poop. Don't get frustrated if one twin may say she has to go just to get attention or just to mimic her twin.

Have a few dry days in a row. After they get the hang of articulating when they have to go and actually go, you can try the undies. Accidents will happen, and what you do about it depends on which twin had one and why. You may want them to help you clean it up, you may want to not make a big deal out of it, you may want to use it as a lecture opportunity, or you may want to have them watch you toss out their soiled prized undies (you can rescue and wash them later) so they won't do it again.

Build the potty into your routine. Once they are in undies, try to put them on the potty as often as possible. This could mean first thing in the morning, before you leave the house for preschool or any morning activities, before you leave preschool to come home, after lunch, before a nap, after a nap, before outside playtime, before dinner, before tub time, and before bed. To help them stay dry at night, you may need to wake them up before you go to bed, and put them on the potty one last time.

Troubleshooting: Training Just One Twin at a Time

Some moms are grateful when twins have staggered readiness, because training one twin at a time seems less physically, emotionally, and logistically daunting. But potty training is time-consuming and requires a good deal of focused attention on the child being trained, so individual training is not without its bumps in the road.

What do you do with Twin B when Twin A is training on the potty? It really depends on how old the twins are when they are training, if there's a safe play area within earshot of the bathroom, and what Twin B's personality is like (docile or wild). If you can, lure Twin B into the loo with some favorite toys and books. You can also lock yourself in the bathroom with both twins until the potty-training session is complete. Another solution: bring a portable potty into the twins' play area and have one sit and train while the other plays. It may be too distracting for Twin A, however, to see Twin B enjoying their regular play environment.

How do you make sure Twin B doesn't feel left out when Twin A is potty-training? As we mentioned earlier, we endorse taking them both shopping with you for potty-training supplies, regardless of their individual degrees of readiness. You can also let Twin B wear undies over a diaper, if that's all Twin B is interested in. We promise that he will not be going off to college like that. If you are incentivizing Twin A with stickers, treats, or special time with Mom or Dad, try giving Twin B incentives to do other things, such as help clean up toys, put her shoes away, or cooperate with what it takes to train Twin A.

Troubleshooting: Training Both Twins Together

Training in tandem can be a relief to moms who prefer to go through the potty-training process once instead of twice. Eager to get it over with in one big swoop and hopeful that the twins will engage in positive peer pressure, these moms limit their time spent as potty coaches. Of course, simultaneous training has its own issues.

Daddy Doc: **Healthy Competition** When it comes to potty training, twins will often spur each other along. Daddy Doc says competition can be a useful thing. When one twin sees the other one getting praise for doing something, frequently that twin will try a little harder. "While punishing one twin for not meeting developmental milestones is inappropriate, rewarding the one who is doing what she is supposed to do is okay," he concludes.

What do you do when Twin A and Twin B want to use the potty at the same time? If it's feasible, we recommend buying two portable potties for your home to help avoid fights over who sits on the toilet and who sits on the potty (the last thing you want to do when urine is about to pour all over your tile floor is referee an argument that could be avoided). The potties with removable buckets (like Baby Bjorn's) are best for quick cleanups, and that way you aren't leaving a mess waiting to be tipped over by eager twins. When they outgrow their portable potties and one of them can't hold the pee while the other is on the bowl, let him or her tinkle on the shower floor or in the tub (or even the sink if you're desperate). It may seem gross, but that's what Lysol is for, and you do what you have to do. If you have twin boys who are comfortable standing and peeing, there's no harm having them share the bowl.

Thrival Tip: We know it is drudgery to clean out portable potties—it might even seem worse than dealing with diapers—but it is for a brief period of time. Very soon the twins will be wiping their own butts, washing their own hands, flushing the toilet, and demanding privacy in the bathroom, so hang in there.

How do you keep things moving when the twins dilly-dally and joke around with each other? Remove all distractions. If they are fooling around with the toilet paper, flushable wipes, or other things in the bathroom, keep them out of reach. Remind them that they are doing potty business and the longer they take, the less time they will have to play and do something fun. Be sure to cut down on your stress about being late for things by padding your schedule. Once training has begun, even with just one twin, give yourself extra time to get them to preschool or other outings.

Potty Training On the Go

When your twins are just getting the hang of wearing underwear, nature may call at the most inopportune times. But take heart, you can thwart on-the-go potty disasters by being prepared.

Bring your stroller if you can still coax them into it. A stroller is a good way to keep one twin from touching all the disgusting things in a public restroom while you are helping the other one on the potty. It's also the fastest way to get the twins to the restroom in a dire situation.

Rework your diaper bag contents. Replace diapers with undies, but keep the wipes, hand sanitzer, plastic bags, and extra clothes. You may need to start carrying extra shoes and socks because pee can dribble down during an accident.

Consider keeping an old beach towel and portable potty in the back of your car. Pulling over on the side of the road or using this in a parking lot is more appealing to some moms than unbuckling both twins from their car seats and walking them into a public restroom. If the other twin suddenly has to go while the portable potty is occupied, encourage him or her to take advantage of the great outdoors.

Twins and Night Training

Some twins may get the hang of staying dry at night soon after they are wearing undies during the day. Others may take weeks or months, or more, to master night dryness. According to Daddy Doc, it's purely a question of physical maturity. He suggests trying to limit late-night drinks, making sure that children use the potty before bed, and being especially careful with sodas, teas, or other caffeinated drinks, which can act as diuretics. He also advocates careful consideration before you abandon nighttime Pull-Ups. Although they may delay nighttime training, as a parent, Daddy Doc knows that it can be very difficult to start the day by changing two beds, which, he says, can "get old very quickly." We concur.

Perhaps the biggest challenge here is when twins wake themselves up in the middle of the night to pee. Personality and maturity come into play: some twins will cry and call out for an escort to the potty, others will sneak into Mom and Dad's room and wake you up for help, and others will pee in the bathroom and hop right back into bed sans parental assistance. If your twins are the loud kind of night wakers, you may feel like you're back in the days of interrupted newborn sleep. If one twin is too disruptive at night, you may want to think about separating their sleeping quarters and moving the night waker closer to a bathroom if at all possible. Another option is rewarding the night waker for doing potty business more quietly.

Thrival Tip: Training accidents happen, sometimes in tandem. Some of our moms have had one or both twins pee or poop in their undies while at a store or at the park. Sure it's embarrassing or frustrating for you and the twins, but it's part of the twin experience, which is mostly enjoyable and fulfilling.

9

OUT AND ABOUT

getting dressed and out the door can be a challenge with young twins in tow. Running to the store for some quick groceries or to the mall to buy a few gifts can turn into an excursion. You're in and out of the house, up and down the stairs, buckling into both sides of the car, reinserting pacifiers or securing hats, folding and unfolding your double stroller . . . it's enough to make you want to stay home. But, of course, that is not always an option. At the very least, you need to head out to show off your adorable babies! When life calls you and your twins out the front door, the best philosophy is to embrace it, and take your show on the road.

Give yourself extra time. It rarely seemed that we could just strap the twins into their car seats and head out the door. Inevitably, someone would poop while we were getting things together, or we'd need to make multiple trips back into the house from the driveway for forgotten items (like the dry cleaning we were all en route to drop off). And wrestling two toddlers into the double stroller, then taking it down to the street from your apartment, probably ends up taking as much time as the Mommy and Me class you're trying to get to. Chances are, you will be late every now and then (or all the time), but integrating back into the world is worth it, so pad your schedule as much as you can and line up babysitting help when there's an appointment you simply must arrive on time for.

Lower your expectations. When you set out to do errands, you can generally expect to get less accomplished than in your previous, pre-twins life. This can be very frustrating because far more planning and strategizing is involved, even for simple outings, than any reasonable person might expect. Cathy sometimes sits in the car in the driveway, children strapped in their car seats, plotting out her local route and getting all relevant paperwork prepared: dry cleaning tickets, money for the drive-through coffee line, checks to deposit at the bank. Making drive-through trips at the beginning or end of your errand route helps minimize the in-and-out-of-the-car-seat process. Two toddlers who are still discovering the wonder of walking can be slow-moving, and keeping two preschoolers from touching everything in the store can be tough, so we've learned to be happy running into two stores rather than the three we had hoped for.

Bring extra stuff. All outings seem to go better when you are properly supplied. Diapers, wipes, changes of clothes, drinks (bottles, sippy cups, or juice boxes), and snacks or some other bribe-related item are all helpful. It's not as though you can't make it work when you are out without your goods, but it does help to minimize the stress when all the stuff you need is right there. Stocking a diaper bag before heading out the door is ideal, but for those who prefer to wing it every once in a while, the car can become your home away from home in case of emergency. You can keep packages of wipes and some diapers tucked into seat storage pockets. Snacks and drinks can be grabbed on the way out the door (though they can also be bought in a pinch). Babies, on the other hand, can't drink from straws, so bottles do need to be prepared ahead of the outing.

Expect attention. One of Cathy's first family outings after the birth of the twins was to the Bronx Zoo in New York. Her husband pushed the infant twins in their stroller and carried their then two-year-old in a backpack. Cathy trailed behind, walking hand in hand with their then four-year-old. By the end of the day, Cathy felt as though her family should be added to the zoo maps as the latest exhibit. People would stop and stare at her husband with three boys in tow, then actually say out loud, after realizing Cathy and their fourth son were part of the group, "Oh my gosh, they have that one, too!" People constantly stopped to ask, "Are they twins?" There's just something about lots of little kids that draws a crowd.

Some moms told us they relish the attention, while others cringe. Even if you usually like it, you might not be so welcoming if you're in a hurry. As one mom said, "All the attention you get when you go out in public makes it difficult to do normal tasks. Going to the grocery store, bank, post office—it's no longer a quick trip." Of course, strangers without twins don't realize all that you had to do to get out the door. We try to be gracious and appreciative of the attention, but we tend to walk and talk.

The twin attraction can also manifest itself when you are dealing with your older children. You might not intend to feature your twins as a sideshow at your older singleton son's kindergarten play, but they naturally draw attention, and for some siblings that can translate into a big distraction. Once in a while, it's nice to lose the group and slip in quietly among the crowd.

Taking that first walk outside with your new babies is one of the best feelings a new mom can experience: a step toward freedom and normalcy. At this stage, proper timing of your outings is a critical factor—it can mean a relaxing walk instead of a run home with two screaming infants. Assuming you're feeding two babies every three hours or so, the time to head out for some fresh air is somewhere between the last burp and the next feeding. In between, you probably need to dress yourself, bundle up your babes, and make sure all your gear is packed. The clock ticks very quickly.

Twin Set Confidential: As tempting as it might be, don't carry two at a time. Cathy was leaving her home with her twins when they were about fifteen months. One was walking, the other not so much. It took an awful long time to get them to cooperate and actually get out the door, so she was eager to get going. To make things easier, she scooped both boys into her arms and started walking down the steps toward her driveway. They were getting heavy by that age, and she had been struggling carrying both boys down the stairs the previous few days. She tripped at the bottom step and easily could have dropped one or both guys on the concrete driveway (she hurt her ankle but they were fine). When you're running late or have had trouble corralling them into coats and shoes to get out the door, it's tempting to simply scoop your babies up, forgoing the stroller or other cumbersome but safe traveling aids. Take it from us, it's not worth it.

Terrific Twinsight: "It's nearly impossible to just run an errand. I have to select which stores I can and can't go to with them and shop accordingly. I can't just run in somewhere."

Out-the-Door Checklist

- ✓ Keys to your home
- ✓ Cell phone (charged)
- ✓ Pacifiers or other soothing tools
- ✓ Comfortable shoes
- ✓ Water for you
- ✓ Clothes or blankets that can be added or removed, depending on the weather

OUT IN PUBLIC

You're not exactly nimble with two babies in bucket car seats, in a stroller, or walking hand in hand. That's why getting your supplies ready before you go out can be extremely helpful. Go through your own mental checklist: Is the stroller in the trunk of the car? Is your diaper bag stocked and ready to go? What are the chances one or both of your twins will melt down before you get home? As a mom of twins, you'll find your equipment choices are not as extensive as those of a mother of one, unless you have another adult with you (for instance, they do make a wearable baby carrier for doubles, but it was not recommended by the moms in our survey). We suggest that for a while at least, you plan to bring your stroller every time you go somewhere. A double stroller is one of the most

A Word on Twins and the Double Stroller

The double stroller is far and away rated the most essential item for moms of twins by the moms we surveyed. The side-by-side option is most popular. Things to consider when making your purchasing decision (and they are not cheap, so it helps to think through these issues): What kind of storage space do you have? Can you lift it in and out of the trunk of your car? Will you be strolling through a mall or on sidewalks, or is it important for you to be able to take your twins for long walks on and off road? Cathy got the Mountain Buggy and still loves it because her twins are comfortable in it even at age two. But she was also lucky enough to receive a hand-me-down Maclaren side-by-side. She used the Mountain Buggy all the time when they were very small; now it's more for walks. The Maclaren is always in the back of the car because it folds up quickly and easily.

important tools a mom of twins can have. One mom said: "A double stroller is huge and difficult to maneuver, but if you ever want to take the babies anywhere by yourself, it is a must." We agree!

That's because the twin challenge comes to a head in public places: they outnumber you. You might feel like it's two against one when they run through the aisles, hide in the clothing racks, or get lost in a crowd (losing sight of one of them for even a second is unbelievably stressful). There's really no way other than a double stroller to ensure you'll have a safe and reliable constraint method. But this can pose challenges, as not every public space is conducive to strollers.

It helps to survey your surroundings in advance. Does your double stroller fit through the door? (A word to the wise: revolv-

When Is It Worth It to Say No?

Ninety-eight percent of the moms we surveyed said they occasionally skip outings because it's just too much work.

Thrival Tips:

- **Try to go out for errands once a day** so you're not getting your twins in and out of car seats or strollers all day long.
- **Teach your toddlers to hold hands in a line** when you're all walking around, especially in parking lots. You can practice this at home, in your driveway, and walking around your block. There should be repercussions if they don't cooperate, though.
- **We recommend putting your twins in a safe place while you get everything ready.** Depending on your living arrangements, moms tell us that sometimes it's easier to strap them into their car seats, then run back into the house to finish gathering all that you need: towels for the beach, hats and mittens to battle the cold, sippy cups or snacks. You can't answer the phone or be engaged for more than half a minute, but it does afford the rare opportunity to carry things using two hands.

ing doors, stairs, and escalators pose some problems.) Is there a clear pathway to walk with your stroller through the aisles? Does your favorite grocery store offer shopping carts with room for two? The grocery store in the town where we live is probably light-years ahead of many others given the concentration of twins in our town, but we've still had to scour the parking lot, twins in tow, looking for a cart with two seats. When it's hot, raining, or we're pressed for time, this frustration can escalate to exasperation.

Despite strategic planning or your best effort to do errands when you can go it alone and leave your twins in the care of a sitter, the day will come when you absolutely must bring your twins with you to shop for that wedding gift off the registry at a china shop. Here are some tips for outings that involve "problem" areas.

- **Near breakables.** Even when they are strapped into their stroller, twin toddlers have amazing reach. Be mindful of where you park your stroller. Could their legs knock a vase off its shelf?
- **Restaurants.** Go early. We typically eat out with our kids at five-thirty, before the adult dinner rush. Make sure they have two high chairs; even family-friendly restaurants might have plenty of booster seats and only one or two wooden chairs.
- **The pharmacy.** The combination of typically being there when one or both of your twins are sick plus the rows and rows of candy and things in tiny boxes makes for less than ideal circumstances. When you and your twins are tired and cranky, things can go wrong. Look into pharmacies that deliver or have drive-through services. In a pinch, the one in our town will send someone out to your car with your prescription, assuming you have a charge account and are parked right out front.
- **House of worship.** Never are our twins as loud as when we take them to church. Try to attend services that are geared toward children, or at least more family-friendly. Alternate going solo with your partner (one of you stays home with the twins) until your twins are old enough to participate or at least sit quietly. The escape option of running out the back carrying one squirmy child is simply not feasible for a parent of twins.

Out-in-Public Checklist

- ✓ Keys to your home
- ✓ Cell phone (charged)
- ✓ Money
- ✓ To-do list
- ✓ Coupons or gift cards
- ✓ Directions
- ✓ The specific items that correspond with your destinations (some examples: party gift, items to return to a store, shoes to be repaired)

Twin Set Confidential: Sometimes we blow

it. We've all pushed our twins too far for the sake of an outing. We've stayed too long at the park and our babies have resorted to screaming to be fed. We've been stuck in traffic and had our toddlers fall asleep for twenty minutes on the way home, just enough time to ruin their afternoon nap. Moms feel so guilty when their twins' routine gets messed up, but it happens. Sometimes it's out of your control; other times it's a result of choices we've made. Regardless, the crying is heartbreaking but not permanently damaging, and you can regain control of the routine the next day.

OUT OF TOWN

Unfamiliar surroundings and a change of pace can be challenging for all kids, and with twins, it can be twice as hard. Cathy's family went on vacation when, at just over two years of age, her twins were old enough to know that a Pack 'n Play isn't as comfortable as their cribs, so what was normally the non-event of putting them to bed became challenging.

New surroundings also pose new challenges: finding a drug-store or doctor, babyproofing, finding your babies' usual milk or toddlers' favorite type of chicken nugget. Again, strategic advance planning is your best tool for ensuring more relaxation than frenzy when on vacation. Truth is, it's tough to just wing it with young twins. They certainly don't need everything to be *exactly* as it is at home, but it creates more work for parents when the routine they rely on for sanity must be adapted. There are steps you can take to minimize the impact unfamiliar surroundings have on your twins and their routine:

- **Choose an environment conducive to young twins.** In many cases, this means renting a house or condo instead of staying in a hotel. Having a kitchen available is extremely helpful for preparing bottles and cups of milk as well as for early-rising twins seeking breakfast.
- **Rent space that does not have multiple levels.** Cathy's husband booked a lovely town house near a ski mountain once when their twins were about ten months old. There were steep stairs and metal furniture. She spent the whole time trying to confine her children to a small corner of the place so they wouldn't fall down the stairs or poke their eyes out on the edge of a modern-style table. Needless to say, it ended up being more work than if they had stayed home.
- **If you do stay in a hotel, consider the impact of two screaming children on your fellow guests.** Where can you go to escape?

Of course, going out of town also introduces the possibility of airplane travel. Cathy avoided the plane altogether until her twins were almost three years of age. The idea of keeping track of four boys under six was just too daunting for her and her husband. But Christina was far more ambitious—she and her husband first flew with all three of their kids together when the twins were six months and big sis was three and a half—and offers some tips for twin air travel:

- **Don't be scared to travel by air when they are still babies.** Yes, it's not fun to schlep two baby buckets on a plane, but baby twins probably are more used to sitting still than toddler twins and they may take better plane naps than toddler or preschool-age twins. Check with your airline to determine their policy on seating when traveling with children under two; some airlines require one adult per child.

- **Check the FAA Web site (faa.gov) to see what you can and can't bring on the plane.** If regulations are really strict, call your airline to see if they can make sure there will be milk, juice, water, or an appropriate snack to give your twins. You'll also need to see what kind of products you can and can't pack in a carry-on diaper bag. Check as much luggage as possible.
- **Check and change diapers before boarding.** Or do potty runs if your twins are training or already trained.
- **Bring your double stroller all the way to the gate.** You'll need it to move the twins and help with all your carry-on stuff.
- **Board the plane with the first group of passengers,** even if that means you have to sit longer before takeoff. Pack quiet toys and books to keep the twins busy. See if you can do man-on-man defense when it comes to sitting on the plane—you take one twin, and Dad takes the other.

Out-of-Town Checklist

✓ Sleep: two Pack 'n Plays with several sheets

✓ Eat: two high chairs or other seating arrangements, bottles, and cups

✓ Portability: probably a stroller and backpacks

✓ Entertainment: a travel DVD player, toys, and books

Twin Transporters

Whether it's traveling across town or across state lines with your twins, different ages require different approaches. Here are some of the pros and cons of each stage.

Newborn to Six Months: The Buckets

Pros: The babies stay where you put them; they are swaddled and cozy; they typically sleep when you're in motion.

Cons: Those buckets are heavy to carry, so you're looking at popping them in a stroller (the double Snap 'N Go is a survey standout). Some places are more stroller-friendly than others.

Six Months to Walking with Confidence

Pros: Babies should be used to sitting cooperatively in the stroller by now, and with toddlers, it's feasible to carry one and hold hands walking with the other.

Cons: If they're in a side-by-side stroller twins may swipe each other's snacks or hurt each other. Or the toddler you are not carrying might have a fit and want you to carry him, too.

Toddlers to Kids

Pros: They are generally stable on their feet and capable of being helpful.

Cons: They can run away! They are far less likely to cooperate with your stroller intentions. And they have the verbal and reasoning skills to scream "Out!" over and over at the top of their lungs.

Part

3

Parenting Twins

over the

Long Haul

10

GOOD HELP

trangers regularly stop us when we're out with our twins in public to say, "I don't know how you do it!" or "Better you than me!" and "Do you have any help?" These encounters remind us that having twins is generally considered not that easy to handle. And it's true, sometimes we *do* need help. It's important to find support when you need it. Here's what helped us secure the best help.

Emotional support. Having at least one person who gets what you are going through and can support you emotionally is essential to your thrival as a mom of twins. It might be a friend you've met through Mothers of Multiples or a mom of twins whom you met at the playground and have traded e-mails with. If you are nursing twins, the support of a local La Leche League group may be what you need. Feeling connected to other moms in the twin community can also be accomplished through reading and responding to blogs on twin-parenting Web sites such as ours, twinsetmoms.com, or through chat rooms. Having a sounding board will let you know that what you are feeling and experiencing as a mom of twins is totally normal.

Hands-on family help. Our survey highlights the important role that family can play in helping out a mom of twins. Family members such as grandmas (our moms are rock stars) are often at least as helpful as paid help in the hours they contribute to the twin cause and the way they help with middle-of-the-night feedings or marathon laundry folding. Friends and neighbors can dig in by carpooling, making meals, and running errands. And last but not least, there's the twins' dad. Overwhelmingly, the moms we talked to are getting the majority of their support from their husbands, whom many call "amazing." Dad can be your best bet and most reliable ally in understanding the work and planning that go into each day of parenting twins. We talked to several dads of multiples to get the inside scoop on how to involve dads and what is going on in their heads and hearts. (Check out the "Dad Support" chapter, page 57, for more.)

What's Your Plan B?

A mom of twins could use some benchwarmers for moments when she's better off doing something solo. Some factors to mull over:

- Are you willing to split the twins up temporarily and have one friend watch one and another friend watch the other?
- Can you deal if their temporary caretaker doesn't stick to your routine?
- How are you going to have to pay this person back? With money, with a favor?
- Can your husband leave work early, go to work late, or take a day off? Or is it smarter to save what you have to/want to do for a weekend day when he's off?

Paid help. Even if you are fortunate enough to have garnered supportive friends and family to assist you in getting through the first few weeks of twin parenthood, you may still feel like it's not enough—and they may have to return to their normal responsibilities. You may want to hire someone to act as your teammate in dealing with the emotional and logistical demands of two children, or to provide you with relief in the form of alone time. Paid backup is worth it when it keeps your twins safe, shaves off layers of your stress, and makes you a better mom.

Thrival Tips: Four Easy Ways to Get More Help

- **Outsource dinner.** Have pizza delivered, buy pre-made meals, collect and use take-out menus.

- **Get your religious community involved.** One of our moms said her church provided her with a dinner every night during her twins' first four weeks. And we could all use extra prayers.

- **Carpool with your neighbors or friends.** If you have other kids who need to be driven around when your twins are babies, take your friends up on their offers. Also, when your twins are older, they may have conflicting activities, and you may need to rely on buddies to get your kids where they need to be.

- **Outsource your chores.** Some dry cleaners, drugstores, and grocery stores deliver. This may be more of a necessity than a luxury for a busy mom of twins. Ask friends and neighbors to refer a laundry service, or search online for a prepared-meals service that delivers to your neck of the woods.

The best things in life are free. For a mom of twins, that means family members and close friends who are willing to pitch in. Here's how to make the most of those kindhearted souls.

Delegate to their strengths and preferences. Sometimes grandparents are more interested in holding and feeding your babies than in folding your laundry. Just let them do what they are happy doing for you. If your uncle is a better cook than diaper changer, point him in the direction of the grocery store and the outdoor grill.

Keep in mind that even those family members who want to help out may not be able to handle twins. It is strenuous, and you more than anyone else should recognize that. If, for example, your mother-in-law tried to help with your twin newborns in the middle of the night and is an exhausted mess the next day, you may want to rethink how you utilize her enthusiasm. She may be better suited to pitching in during the day, which won't seem as long to you if you have a rested helper. Some family members may own up that they can't hack it and suggest alternative roles for themselves, or even that maybe someone else should help you instead of them. In some families this kind of honesty is rare, so do your best to appreciate it and come up with a Plan B.

Routinely assess your needs and the twins' evolution. You may not be able to count on an older relative helping out when your twins are active toddlers, bolting in two different directions. If you have no choice, consider running errands or grabbing a bite to eat only when the twins are napping or down for the night.

Twin Set Confidential: Grumpy New Moms

Our survey respondents said the first several weeks of twin parenting, which we call the Big Blur, are the hardest. To be honest, sometimes the first few weeks brought out the worst in us. At our low points, we were hypersensitive to any suggestions from family members, resentful that people weren't physically helping us enough, and angry that we had to tell people what to do to help because they couldn't figure it out on their own. We had enough to manage trying to care for the twins and our other kids, didn't we? Why did we have to manage the grown-ups who were supposed to be helping us, too? Eventually, things settled down. Some rest and alone time worked wonders on our dispositions. And coming up with specific ways that people could help made a huge difference, too.

Think of little things that others can do to help you out big-time. We had mom friends watch our twins in the car so we could quickly run into preschool and pick up our singletons and the friend's kid, too. We also called each other when we were doing Costco, Babies R Us, or grocery store runs to see if the other needed anything. We had friends who were nice enough to invite our older kids over on play dates so that we'd have just the twins to deal with for a while. We asked friends for help with our bigger kids when our twins got sick (and of course, returned the favor when they needed help).

Appreciate all the little things they do. Say thanks often so friends and family feel motivated to keep helping.

Strategically schedule guest visits. If you can swing it, ask adoring fans to come over right before feedings, so they can hold and feed a baby while you chitchat. Or invite someone over to cover for you when the twins are napping so you can get out.

Terrific Twinsight: "I don't know how I survived.
The floors went unwashed. I often didn't shower. I very rarely cooked dinner. My husband ran out of underwear and clean socks on a regular basis. But these things took the backseat to my triplet girls. If they were clean, fed, and happy, then that is all that mattered."

USING PAID HELP WHEN YOU NEED IT MOST

You can ease the financial strain by only using paid childcare when you really need it. For example, it was most important for Cathy to keep some things regular for her two older boys after her twins were born. That meant continuing to be on the go, attending their kiddie music or gymnastic classes and participating in group play dates. These environments (noisy, germy, and chaotic) are not always a great idea for newborns. To help manage the divergent needs of her two sets of boys, and with the absence of family nearby, she bulked up on help during her twins' first year. When they were toddlers and she was working at home, she cut way back, and counted on their regular midday nap to get stuff done.

How Much Paid Help Do Moms Have?

Forty percent of the moms we surveyed said they currently have no paid help.
Eight percent said they have less than five hours.
Eleven percent said they have five to ten hours.
Ten percent said they have ten to twenty hours.
Sixteen percent said they have twenty to forty hours.
Fifteen percent said they have more than forty hours.

Talk to local Mothers of Multiples Club members or friends with twins (or at least two close-in-age children) to get a gauge on what child care costs you might expect for your twins (check out your club's Web site or newsletter for leads on nannies, baby nurses, and babysitters). We have a list of considerations to help you plan and budget for when you may need paid help the most.

- **Twins' ages.** According to the moms we surveyed, they needed the most help during the first four months of their twins' lives, and again when twins were around eighteen months to two or three years old. But we were happy to know that a whopping 68 percent of our respondents said they had the help they needed during these two long age ranges. This high rate can probably be attributed to advance planning and being creative in seeking help (keeping names and numbers of potential helpers that you meet or hear of in your travels) and proactive in following up with folks who offer it.
- **Twins' health.** Unfortunately, national statistics reveal that about 50 percent of twins end up in the NICU. And in many cases, one remains in the NICU when the other is at home. Having a plan in place can make things much less stressful in the event that one or both of your twins needs special care. Going forward, twins with severe special needs or health issues may require more at-home care than you were counting on. Also, since all twins get sick at some point, it's essential to have backup to call if you need to rush one to the doctor or hospital. Make sure your backups know that you consider them to be emergency contacts and that they think they can handle the responsibility beforehand.
- **Your health.** When we get really sick or have suffered an injury, we feel stress at its peak. We know we need to get rest, but we are consumed by thoughts of the twins and our other kids, and of all we have to do. If the twins are in good hands, that's one less worry and more beneficial rest time for you. Speaking of not feeling well, you may get pregnant again when the twins are little. Some pregnant

moms are restricted in terms of physical activity, so help may become vital.

- **Times of day.** You may be able to find a baby nurse to help in the wee hours, a sitter to come over to help from dinner through tuck-in time, or a drop-off place for two hours every morning so you can exercise and run quick errands. Think about when you are the most tired, stressed, or in need of time to yourself. One mom said she'd love some help getting her toddlers dressed and out the door in the winter. Think about the timing of other responsibilities in your life, such as when you need to drive your other children places, your job hours, your husband's hours, and when the gym or grocery store are less crowded.

- **Your lifestyle.** If you plan on continuing to be very social after you have twins, you may want to make sure you have reliable babysitting, so you can go on dates with your spouse or out to dinner with friends. Many moms of twins don't leave home at night until the twins are tucked in. This way, they can enjoy their time outside the home knowing their twins are dreaming sweetly.

- **Your climate.** If the weather is rotten (freezing cold, pouring rain, or boiling hot), it's no fun to get the twins in and out of the car or buildings by yourself. Also, if one twin is sick and better off staying home in extreme weather, you can divvy up the twins with a helper.

WHAT TYPE OF PAID HELP IS BEST FOR YOU?

There are lots of child care options for infant, toddler, and preschool-age twins. We'll break it all down for you, plus resources and info from our survey moms.

Type of help: Baby nurse
Twins' age: Birth to six months

How to find one: Word of mouth, twins club, babynurse.com, or gentlehandschildcare.com

Pros: A baby nurse is essentially an experienced nanny with extensive training and certifications in newborn care that include CPR and infant massage. (A baby nurse is not a licensed medical professional.) The focus of a baby nurse is on the twins and helping them establish sleeping and eating patterns. This option is popular with moms of twins who need help breast-feeding two newborns while recovering from a C-section (with restrictions on lifting and taking the stairs). About 32 percent of our respondents used a baby/night nurse, most (45 percent) for six weeks or less. Almost 38 percent said they couldn't have done it without her, and almost 30 percent said it was a smart long-term investment because a successful routine was established. One mom said, "It was the best $10,000 we ever spent." You can hire one for as little (one night, here and there) or as long (months at a time) as you like. A baby nurse should help with complete care of babies, and may help with household laundry or caring for older siblings.

Cons: This is a costly option. One mom said it cost her about $270 a night. The Web site gentlehandschildcare.com says you can expect to pay upward of $250 a day for a live-in baby nurse who provides twenty-four-hour care or about $19 to $35 an hour for à la carte help. Only 2 percent of those respondents who used a baby nurse said it wasn't worth the money. Consider that it is another person to manage, when you may already be mentally maxed out or just tired of giving orders. About 5 percent said accommodating the nurse was more stressful than helpful, and almost 4 percent had trouble handing over the babies to her care. In some cases, your husband or your family may not get along with her or agree with her scheduling practices. A baby nurse in your home requires a serious comfort level for both you and your husband. Remember, you'll probably be at your weakest, so make sure the effort of finding, paying, and accommodating someone is worth it.

Type of help: *Doula*
Twins' age: Before, during, and after their birth
How to find one: Dona International (www.dona.org)
Pros: A doula focuses on the emotional support and physical comfort of a mom before, during, and after childbirth. To be a doula, you need to complete a two-year certification process that includes classes on childbirthing, midwifery, and breast-feeding. A doula can accompany you at the birth of your twins, and she can also come to your home after they are born to care for you during your recovery for a prearranged period of time (days or weeks). She'll help to educate you about breast-feeding and will help care for the babies. Some doulas may assist with running errands and doing chores that pertain to you and your twins. This could be heavenly for a mom who's had a C-section or is breast-feeding.
Cons: It's another person to manage (a sort of wife for you). It can also be costly. According to doula.com, it can cost about $300 to $1,000 to hire a doula for prenatal time, on-call time, childbirth time, and postpartum time. Ask a potential doula about her experience and what services she will provide during her visits with you to see if you think it's worth it. To find a less expensive doula, you can consider working with a doula in training or ask your local hospital if they offer doula services for free. Another consideration is asking your insurance company if they will cover some or all of the cost.

Type of help: *Lactation consultant*
Twins' age: Before your twins are born to learn how to prepare to nurse them and then again when they are newborns or whenever you or they are having difficulty nursing

How to find one: The hospital where you gave birth, your pediatrician, your OB/GYN, La Leche League (lllusa.org)

Pros: Your insurance might help pay for this. Many hospitals offer nursing consultations while you're there (at no additional charge) or even have nursing groups that meet for free after you're discharged. Many consultants will make themselves available to you by phone. Some will even come to your home, so they can see where you nurse the twins, help you get more comfortable with propping and pillows, show you different holds (simultaneous and individual) to decrease pain, help each baby latch on better, and help any breast infections or clogged milk ducts heal. They may even make special product recommendations, such as nursing pillows designed for moms of twins. It may take more than one visit to improve your nursing experience. Frequent phone consults with an expert might provide the confidence you need to keep going.

Cons: Once you are home with your twins, you may find it difficult to get back to the hospital's lactation group meetings or frustrating to get the hospital's lactation consultant on the phone. You may need to research finding one who can visit you at home, and that's going to take time and energy that you may not have.

Type of help: *Live-out babysitter*
Twins' age: From birth on
How to find one: Word of mouth, twins club, sittercity.com, craigslist.com (posting is free), local university students, child care resource and referral agencies (childcareaware.org)

Pros: You can keep your twins in the comfort of their own surroundings. You may trust the sitter enough to let him or her take your twins for long walks, play with them outside, or drive them to activities when they are older. A sitter may give you the flexibility you want to work from home, go to the gym, run errands, or do things for yourself. You're also not locked into a contract, so you can change your babysitter as your twins develop if the sitter isn't capable of rising to the new standards. You may be able to arrange a sharing agreement with a friend of yours. When twins are sick, the sitter can stay home with the healthy one, so you only have to take the sick child to the doctor.

Cons: Since you aren't locked into a contract, you might get hit with a sudden rate hike, or your beloved sitter may get poached by another family. Sometimes sitters lose their luster after getting too comfortable with the job, and it can be hard for a mom to dispense constructive criticism due to the very personal nature of the working relationship. If your sitter has other jobs, they may take priority over your needs or limit her flexibility when you need her most (when you're sick, when the twins are). Some sitters may not be able to hack the demands of watching twins, especially if there is no downtime on the job (there is laundry or housecleaning to do during the twins' nap time).

Must Love Multiples

Who is the perfect caregiving match to hire for your twins? Here are some personal and professional backgrounds that might be a plus.

- Ex-teachers are used to commanding a room rather than singling out one child.
- People who grew up in a big family will be used to noise, chaos, mess, and constant activity.
- A retiree with a gentle soul might not get fazed by two screaming babies and would be more willing to rock your babies in a chair all day, if need be.
- A nurse, lifeguard, or EMT is used to preparing ahead to avoid danger and might have excellent common sense, disaster aversion skills, and first aid knowledge.
- A mother of older, school-age kids is used to multitasking and staying calm under pressure.

Checklist: What to Ask When Interviewing a Prospective Caregiver

After you have checked references, you may feel comfortable interviewing a candidate at your home, so he or she can see what kind of systems you have in place to care for and entertain the twins and what the twins are like. Someone with tons of babysitting experience may never have dealt with twins, and it may be a real eye-opener. Questions to incorporate in your discussion might include:

- Do you have any twin experience, personally or professionally?
- What will you do when both twins are sick, crying, naughty, or whining?
- How do you feel about following our family's schedule?
- Are you willing to do laundry and light cleaning when the twins are napping?
- How will you feel about working in a home where one or both of the parents are around a lot?
- Can you juggle caring for our other children as well?
- Do you have children or anyone else who's dependent on you that might impact your ability to get to work?
- Do you have any personal requests that might be difficult for us to meet?
- Do you have any personal relationships that are challenging and might impact your job performance or attitude?
- Do you have any transportation challenges?
- Can you drive and swim? Do you know CPR? If not, would you be willing to take a course?
- How flexible is your schedule? What kind of hours do you want/need?
- How are you to be paid? Can we expect a rate increase anytime soon?
- How long were you at your last job? Why did you leave that job?
- Do you understand that drinking, smoking, and drug use are forbidden on the job?

Type of help: Live-in nanny
Twins' age: From birth on
How to find one: eNannySource.com, nannypoppins.com, childcareaware.org
Pros: If you hire one without the help of an agency, you can set the ground rules for hours, expectations, and how flexible you want things to be. She can help with the twins, older siblings, cooking, cleaning, and laundry. A nanny may be a better value per hour than

a live-out sitter (don't forget to factor in room and board). Also, since a nanny lives with you, he or she will really understand how the twins operate, so handing off the two kids to the nanny's care should be easy. Some moms hire a nanny just for the summer, when they know they'll be out more with the twins and could use the extra support. Many college students do this as a way to experience life in a different part of the United States. Generally, caretakers who live with you afford far more flexible schedules than those who live out. Plus, you are the top priority.

Cons: If you use an agency, there may be strict parameters for the total amount of hours worked each week and time off that don't jive with your needs. It can be really weird to get used to having someone live in your house and gradually become part of your family. You may be living in tight quarters and sacrifice some privacy for some sanity.

Type of help: *Au pair*

Twins' age: An au pair (a foreign national granted temporary stay by the U.S. State Department) can't legally be left alone to care for a baby less than twelve weeks of age. But you can hire one to start before your twins are three months old to begin training him or her while you are home.

Do You Need to Run a Background Check?

Use your common sense, your gut instinct, and the information you have garnered to determine if you need to check a candidate's background further in order to keep your twins safe and well cared for. You can run a social security number trace, check DMV records, and search credit reports to verify a person's name and address and driving experience (if they have a DUI, several speeding tickets, dozens of unpaid parking tickets). If you decide that you want to look into whether a candidate has a criminal record, you can visit babysafeamerica.com, babysitters.com, crimcheck .com, integctr.com, findoutnow.net, or nannybackgroundcheck.com. Call your local police department and ask them for tips on screening a potential caregiver.

Checklist: What to Ask When Checking References for a Potential Caregiver

Regardless of what type of paid help you consider, you should check at least three recent references for a potential candidate. Take notes when checking references, listen to what is not said about a candidate, and remember to ask these questions.

- How did you meet the candidate? How would you rate your relationship with him or her?
- How long did the candidate work for you? Why did the job end?
- Is the candidate extremely patient and good at multitasking? Does the candidate stay calm under pressure and have strong common sense?
- What do you think the candidate will do when both twins are crying, whining, or fighting?
- Did the candidate follow your family's schedule?
- How do you think the candidate will discipline the twins?
- Can the candidate watch two or more active children and keep them entertained and safe?
- How did the candidate feel about working if you were home a lot?
- Did the candidate have any personal requests that were difficult for you to meet?
- Does the candidate have any outside relationships that are questionable or challenging, any personality quirks that are a source of concern, any confidence or safety issues, or any transportation challenges?
- Does the candidate have any special skills, such as cooking, driving, or swimming?
- Did you let the candidate drive your children? Did the candidate drive your car or his or her own car? Did you insure the candidate under your policy?
- How did you pay the candidate? Were there frequent rate increases?
- Did you ever suspect that the candidate drank alcohol, smoked, or used drugs on the job?
- Have you met any of the candidate's friends or family? What are they like?
- What are your recommendations for establishing a healthy working relationship with the candidate?

How to find one: There are lots of au pair agencies out there. Find one with au pairs already present in your community and talk to their host families about their experiences.

Pros: The rules governing hiring a foreign au pair are overseen by the U.S. Department of Labor and the Bureau of Educational and Cultural Affairs, so there's no guesswork involved in terms of how long they can work for you, how much you pay them, and what their vacation requirements are. Au pairs are generally economically efficient: you get a lot of hours of care for less than you'd pay a nanny or live-out sitter. There is a screening process that au pair companies do, along with providing references. You are in control of the schedule and can change it every week, according to your needs. An au pair can offer you lots of flexibility to adapt to the twins' changing needs.

Cons: They are generally young and inexperienced with twins. It may be challenging because of the social lives they enjoy when they are not on duty. An au pair may experience culture shock or intense homesickness. The language barrier may be hard to break. They may not take the job seriously and may decide to find another host family if they don't like yours.

Type of help: *Day care*
Twins' age: Depends on the facility
How to find one: Start with the National Child Care Information Center (nccic.org). Each state has different rules and regulations when it comes to day care centers.

Pros: Some parents of twins feel a day care facility is better equipped to deal with multiples because they are used to juggling kids of similar ages and developmental phases. Your twins may assimilate well because they are used to sharing *your* attention. You might find one near your office, so you can visit your twins on your coffee or lunch break.

Cons: Exposing your twins to a bunch of other kids means they may get sick a lot. Our working moms said they had a really hard time finding a day care that would reserve two infant spots in advance or had two baby openings after the twins were born. Your twins may not get the same attention that a dedicated sitter may provide.

Type of help: *Preschools and camps*
Twins' age: Many preschools and camps start around age two. Potty training may be a requirement for a program meant for three-year-olds and up.
How to find one: Local newspapers and phone books, word of mouth
Pros: Your twins are in a stimulating environment and able to socialize with other kids their age. This may give them an opportunity to spread their wings.
Cons: If your twins are really attached to each other, they may have a hard time mixing with other kids. Or one twin might be ready to socialize and the other not. Preschools, camps, and drop-off activities can get pricey, especially when you are paying double. Some places offer a sibling discount, so ask.

Type of help: *Drop-off babysitting center*
Twins' age: Depends on the facility
How to find one: Local gyms, places of worship, YMCA or YWCA
Pros: You get to do the things that are important to you, such as praying, taking classes, or working out, with peace of mind because your babies are in the same building as you are.
Cons: If your twins don't go to this place often, the transition may be rocky. Or you may be uncomfortable because you're not familiar with the child care provider on duty.

Twincidentals: When Child Care Providers Play Favorites

It's natural that your twins have two distinct personalities and that one of them may be more appealing for your sitter, nanny, or preschool teacher than the other. Twins are not the same as two classmates—they live in relation to each other and tend to be hyperaware of the need to maintain equality between them. If you feel one twin is getting special attention to the dismay of the other, you may need to ask the child care provider to be more aware of how he or she interacts with the twins. It's the caregiver's job to make both feel comfortable and cared for.

Type of help: *Mother's helper*

Twins' age: From infancy on

How to find one: Word of mouth, school job boards, your neighborhood

Pros: This is an inexpensive, old-fashioned approach to getting a little extra help while still running the show. Your mother's helper could be your neighbor, your older daughter, or your nephew. Regardless, you may be pleasantly surprised by how mature and capable a nine-year-old seems compared to your exuberant sixteen-month-old dynamos. A sitter age eleven to fifteen can take the Babysitter's Training Course through your local Red Cross (see redcross.org for more info).

Cons: Your mother's helper may need more help from you than you're getting from him or her. Since they are young, immaturity when it comes to managing a job might come into play. For example, they may not have a handle on their availability but need to check with their parents, and you might find yourself competing for attention with social engagements, sports, and midterms. Don't count on a mother's helper to do too much, such as heavy lifting, changing diapers, cleaning up dirty messes, or monitoring potty training twins.

Things You May Need to Provide for Your Child Care Provider

- **Twin manual.** Fill a few pages of a notebook with details on each twin's likes, dislikes, habits, medication, allergies, etc. Leave room for your caregiver to jot down questions or notes about the twins (who pooped, napped, snacked, etc.).
- **Driver's insurance.** You may have to cover your nanny, au pair, or sitter under your policy if he or she is driving your car.
- **Cell phone.** Find a plan with limited minutes and set ground rules for the phone's use by your caregiver.
- **Phone card.** If your caregiver's family is abroad, this may be an economic alternative to buying him or her a cell phone.
- **Computer access.** E-mailing is cheaper than talking on a phone. Set rules on downloading, surfing, and so on. Think about upgrading the security on your computer. Or give your caregiver time to go to your public library to use the computers there.

Type of help: Cleaning service/person

Twins' age: From birth on

How to find one: Word of mouth, friends with clean homes, mollymaid.com or merrymaid.com

Pros: You will have plenty of cleaning up to do yourself with all the messes that involve your twins, so it's great to have a professional take care of the heavy-duty vacuuming, dusting, and floor washing. Decide how often you want your cleaning person or service to come and what kind of cleaning supplies they'll use. You may want them to change the bed linens and fold laundry.

Cons: Your twins' nap schedule may evolve and become tricky to work around with a cleaning crew, as opposed to one cleaner, in the home. If it is a crew, you may not be guaranteed to have the same people show up and work each time.

Balancing a job and family is difficult: It's stressful to be productive at work and to carve out time for your twins. (See our "Mom Care" chapter on page 35 for tips on making time to care for yourself. Yes, *you*!) More than 34 percent of the moms we surveyed work outside of the home full or part time, and 10 percent work at home. The majority of these moms said it is much more difficult to find qualified and affordable child care solutions when you have twins. Many moms told us they elected not to return to their jobs after the birth of their twins because the double day care fee or higher babysitter rates made it financially unappealing.

Making the Tax Laws Work for You

Check out irs.gov to discover the latest tax breaks for working parents with child care expenses. If you and your husband work, you may qualify to save hundreds or thousands of dollars a year.

"No one would watch my twins," one mom said. "All the day care centers said, 'It's so hard, we don't know how you do it.'" Rather than get defeated by the challenge of finding good care, here's how the working moms we surveyed got creative:

- **Changed hours.** One mom took the second shift at the hospital where she works so her husband can care for their twins in the evening. She picks up more hours working every other weekend when he's home.

- **Traded places.** One mom has a work-at-home husband who works way less than he used to, as he now takes care of the twins while she's back at work.
- **Shared nannies.** Part-time working moms split nannies with friends.
- **Supported Grandma.** One mom hired a babysitter to help her mother (the twins' grandma) watch her twins and her sister's kids.

11

BONDS AND RIVALRIES

One of your greatest privileges as a parent will be nurturing your twins' special bond with each other. Some days you may want to ensure that they get quality time together or that you deal with them evenhandedly so they don't resent each other. Other days, you may wonder if they'll ever get along because they are so different or too similar. To guide a set of twins through the emotional ups and downs of having a constant companion is rigorous but truly rewarding. On the tougher days with your two, you may lack the patience or confidence you need to deal with their dynamic. That's when you have to remember to trust your instincts, because you know your twins better than anyone else—well, except maybe each other.

TWIN BONDING: THE CUTE THINGS TWINS DO

If you look more closely at your sonogram photos, you may realize that your twins began bonding in your womb. Soon after they were born, one twin may have been comforted when the other was placed close by. When it comes to adorable twin bond phenomena, almost half of our survey moms said they've witnessed their babies holding hands, and almost 20 percent have had an earful of twin-speak, the secret language that twins can share. (You know you're hearing twin-speak if it sounds like gobbledygook that they find hilarious but you don't understand at all.) Many moms told us that one twin regularly sneaks out of bed at night and cozies up with his or her twin. In fact, 40 percent of our survey respondents report being amazed by their twins' bond. Moms also shared three favorite twin-bonding moments: seeing their twins make sure the other gets his or her fair share, watching their twins sticking up for each other, and hearing their double darlings tell people that they are twins.

So what makes some twins so tight? Twins love each other as built-in childhood playmates, trusted advocates, sounding boards, best friends forever, perhaps even soul mates. In some cases, as 14 percent of the moms who answered our survey said, you may even feel like a third wheel once in a while around your twins. If your twins are identical, experts tell us that they share genetic personality traits, meaning they will most likely have similar interests, habits, and temperaments. Fraternals may not have as much DNA in common as identicals and may have drastically different personalities, quirks, likes, and dislikes, but maybe those differences complement each other and balance each other out.

Giving twins space to bond. As a parent of twins, you may feel an unspoken pressure that your babies should grow up being intensely emotionally connected. If your babies don't enjoy co-sleeping, simultaneous nursing, or playing with each other, you may wonder why not. Our survey showed that 25 percent of moms have been disappointed, at least once in a while, by the lack of closeness between their twins. From our experiences, we urge you not to give up on the power of two. Rather, give your twins the space to find their way to each other and figure it out.

Cathy wasn't so sure that this was going to happen for her boys. They started out in the hospital sleeping in separate cribs and as they got older still seemed to prefer being alone, with a parent, or with their older brothers rather than each other. The indifference almost—*almost*—made her long for a battle to break out just so they'd at least be acknowledging each other. They really didn't start engaging each other until they were about eighteen months old. It was a huge relief to Cathy, who reports that as their social skills progress and continue to mature, so does their friendship and genuine interest in each other.

The Boy/Girl Twin Bond

For parents of boy/girl twins, it can be a dream come true to get the son and daughter you've always dreamed of with one pregnancy (how efficient!). But Christina knows that having one boy and one girl of the same age can be complicated. Here's how the moms we surveyed experienced it:

Seventy-two percent said boy/girl twins have more divergent interests than same-sex twins.

Forty-five percent said having a twin of the opposite gender has affected their twins, compared to if they had been the same gender.

One-third said their boy/girl twins have different friends.

Forty-six percent said their boy/girl twins are as competitive with each other as same-sex twins.

Ninety-four percent said their boy/girl twins have a harder time sharing.

Ninety-five percent said their boy/girl twins understand each other as well as same-gender twins.

Christina's concern was that her boy/girl twins were so different that they couldn't possibly end up being twin-tight. But her three-year-old twins can often be found hiding behind the family room couch with a blanket on their heads, cracking each other up by making up silly names for each other and funny new words. It's impossible to get their attention when they are in this twin world. It's hard to imagine that she was once so worried that they wouldn't be close!

Fostering the twin connection. In addition to patiently observing your twins' discoveries, there are ways to help them appreciate each other.

- **Keep them on the same routine.** They will see each other more often, have the same playtime, and be more likely to be in well-rested, happy, playful moods at the same time.
- **Have them share a room.** Some moms say their baby twins get used to hearing each other cry pretty quickly and learn to sleep through it. The payoff can be huge: you get to hear their intimate crib chat over the baby monitor.
- **Give them twin time.** Your babies need time alone with you, but they also will benefit from time alone with each other, just relaxing and playing without any distractions.
- **Take them to special places together.** When you can manage it, consider signing up for a Mommy and Me class so you and the twins can share a positive, stimulating experience together on a regular basis. (Check whether the teacher will help you handle one of the twins while you are with the other.)
- **Let them choose or make something special for each other.** Exchanging simple homemade birthday cards or dollar treats from the candy store can be worth a fortune in happy memories.

The importance of fostering your twins' individualities was a recurring theme among our survey respondents. Giving each twin a strong sense of self is a powerful way to prepare them to make decisions and to cope with life's hard knocks. Making this a parenting priority is challenging—we are so used to getting through the daily routine by treating the twins as a set. As twins age and negotiating fairness becomes their obsession, you may constantly think in terms of two at a time. But as our Mommy Doc says, "An important but difficult lesson is that twins don't have to be treated equally at all times."

Many parents of twins, caught up in the excitement of a twin pregnancy, bestow upon their children matching names and go to great lengths to dress them in matching outfits (hard to resist because they do look super-cute). We have all forced the twin dynamic in one way or another. But it's not always a good thing. As one mom put it poignantly, "You don't want to walk through life as someone's shadow. Nobody does." A second mom told us that, in hindsight, she wished she had not fostered that type of dynamic. Another drawback of the twin dynamic, according to almost half our survey moms, is that they experience strong feelings of guilt because "I fear I'm not giving enough to each child." One mom said, "It's tough making alone time for one twin. If I try, it's stressful because the other one is crying for me." When you have other kids to parent, too, it's even more challenging. One of our moms confesses, "I have an older child who was only two and a half when the twins were born. Dividing myself three ways and feeling like I am there for all of my children has always been my biggest stress."

But take heart—moms of twins are great at making the best of difficult circumstances. No matter what you named your twins, what they wear, or whom your twins will be up against in life, you can arm each of them with solid self-esteem. Try some of these ideas for making each twin feel special:

- **Refer to them by their first names.** Don't speak of them collectively as "the twins."
- **Give them their own birthday cakes** if they share the party.
- **Give them different gifts.** Also let friends and family know if you'd like them to have individual gifts for birthdays, holidays, and special occasions (13 percent of our moms say this is important).
- **Take some pictures of them without their twin.** Do this solo and with family and friends.
- **Acknowledge individual achievements.** Almost 70 percent reward just one twin when he or she performs well.
- **Sign them up for different activities.** Maybe you can do one activity with both of them (for twin bonding), and find a second activity that suits their individual interests. This may require you to get a sitter for the twin who's not going to an activity.
- **Do chores with only one twin in tow.** Visiting the car wash can be fun for a kid, and the travel and cleaning time allow for some special time together. Also consider divvying up the chores with Daddy so each twin gets alone time with each parent.
- **Bathe them solo.** Put one in a safe place with a book. Bath time can go from stressfest to relaxing and fun when each child gets a turn soaking in a parent's attention along with the soapy bubbles.
- **Provide extra snuggles on sick days.** If one is stuck home from school due to an injury or illness, see it as a chance to cherish him or her. Your attention will have incredible healing power, too.
- **See the sweeter side of night waking.** If your twins are normally good sleepers, try to view an occasional middle-of-the-night disruption as a chance to give them an extra hug and lullaby. (If they're regular night wakers, check out our "Sleep Strategies" chapter on page 93.)

Terrific Twinsight: "I stress the need for their pre-school teachers to learn as much about the twins as they can so that they can tell them apart. My twins are two and a half years old and love to trick people into thinking they are talking to the 'other' twin. They like to play 'tricky trick to you' to people."

- **Call in the reinforcements.** If you can't be there for extra-special time due to work or other circumstances, line up Grandpa or another loved one to smother each twin with TLC.

For parents of identical twins it can be challenging to help teachers, caregivers, and other parents and children tell your kids apart.

Twincidentals: Matching Wardrobes, Dueling Opinions

How you want to dress your twins can be an emotionally charged issue. Some days you may want to proudly advertise the twinness; on others you may want to play it down. Sometimes you may not even realize what they are wearing—you just pulled from the clean clothes pile! If you are more inclined to enjoy the twinship while they are still little, it may be heartbreaking when one twin vocalizes a desire to be independent and not match his or her twin anymore. Other twins may be split in their opinions: one may like it, the other may not. This can be hurtful for the enthusiastic twin. You may be able to smooth things out by dressing them in similar styles, just in different colors or patterns. Bottom line: take lots of pictures of your twins when they are babies and wearing exactly what you want!

Twin Set Confidential: Twenty-seven percent

of moms with identicals admit they've confused their own twins once in a while.

(One-fifth of our survey moms have identical twins; in 2004, less than 1 percent of births were identical twins.) Some fraternal twins look so similar that they are called "mirror twins." Even if you don't think your twins—identical or fraternal—look alike, others may still get confused. Here are the most popular distinguishing strategies used by moms:

- Take the initiative to introduce each twin by name—over and over, again and again.
- Dress them in different outfits and colors. Pick one or two colors for each twin and stick with them all the time.
- Give the twins different hairstyles.
- Put different color earrings on girls.
- Point out distinctions like who has the raspier voice, the birthmark on one cheek, and so on.

Perhaps the funniest tip: "Mine wear different color sneakers so when they are running away and I am behind them I can scream the right name."

THE TWIN BOND GONE WILD

Even though twins can be extremely close and affectionate, the bond can have a downside. Some twins cause trouble together, and it's twice as hard to get them to stop making mischief because it's like dealing with a mini mob. One mom reveals that she's stressed out by "the constant trouble they get into because they are showing off for each other." One mom of triplets tells us that she often feels ganged up on by her kids. It's disheartening when one twin teaches the other bad behavior. It's like having a mischievous play date over whom you can't send back home after a couple of hours.

Short of wearing a referee shirt and blowing a whistle, there are things you can do to help your twins act less naughty and more nice. The moms we surveyed say that consistency and follow-through are the best ways to get a handle on raucous twins. If you say you are going to put one or both in time-out, do it; if you say you are going to take away their favorite toys, do it, even if that means you have to listen to two sets of lungs scream. Trust us; it's worth it to regain control. And you can be sure the twins are keeping score. If you are harsh on one and not the other for the same transgression, the more severely reprimanded one will surely call you out for not being fair. That's why more than 90 percent of the moms we surveyed stick to one set of rules for both twins to follow.

Sometimes things between the twins get a little too physical and biting, hitting, or kicking occurs. Sixty percent of the moms we surveyed said they have been shocked by the way their twins have hurt each other. Biting can start at a young age, when twins are toddlers who get frustrated and can't verbalize their feelings. The hitting and kicking may come into play when twins are older and capable of using words but not capable of self-control when their twin is ticking them off. If one or both of your twins bites,

Terrific Twinsight: "If one is doing something wrong and I speak with him about it, the other one sticks up for him. I have come to realize that separation is key when discipline is necessary."

take heart. Mommy Doc says, "I think smaller incidents like biting are more common in twins. I think that twins will act out their frustrations on each other. You have two children forced to interact with each other socially when they are not developmentally ready to move beyond parallel play."

Now that you know that biting may be a twin thing, what can you do to get it to stop? Christina felt that her twins' pediatrician gave her good advice when her son bit his twin sister a couple of times. First, tend to the hurt twin. Then look the twin biter in the eye while holding his chin in your hand and say, "No biting." Next, put the biter in his crib or on his bed for several minutes. When you retrieve the biter, make sure he seems contrite and give him a final on-the-spot reminder about not biting. During routine checkups at the pediatrician, Christina had the doctor reinforce her no-biting campaign by chatting with her son about being a big boy and not hurting his sister. A zero-tolerance policy seemed to help stop the biting.

Naughty twins on the loose. Twins are so used to confinement (waiting for their bath in a crib, being strapped in a stroller while Mommy quickly weeds the garden outside, and playing in a play yard) that when restraints are removed, mostly around age two and a half, some go bonkers and can't handle the freedom. From our experience, it's best to gradually phase out any restraints rather than do it all at once. For example, you may be able to take them out of high chairs during mealtime when they are two and a half, but you may want to keep up the gate that will keep them from running into the living room with tomato sauce on their hands. When her twins turned three, Christina tried switching them from car seats with a harness to car seats with a cross-lap belt. They kept unbuckling the seat belts themselves at inopportune times and climbing all over the car. Luckily for Christina, the old car seats were resting in the garage and were reemployed after about a week of twin nonsense. Six months later, the cross-lap belt seats were successfully reintroduced.

Secrets of minimizing sibling rivalry. Even if you staunchly defend your twins against comparisons or labels from the outside world and work hard at respecting their individuality, your twins might still develop a problematic sense of competition with each other. To reduce the innate competition, a mom can try these strategies.

- **Praise one twin for a job well done, and throw a verbal bone to the other one as well.** Remember, praising is not the same as rewarding.
- **Teach the twins to share toys and to take turns.** Make sure they understand that some things (such as the stuffed animal they sleep with every night) retain "special" status and are non-negotiable.
- **Have balanced play dates.** Do your best to make sure one twin isn't moping around because he is bored or left out. On some days, that might mean you have one friend over for each twin.
- **Make sure the number and size of gifts from you are about equal.** If one twin gets a new bike as a birthday gift and the other gets a hand-me-down from an older sibling, all heck can break loose.
- **Let them start working out fights on their own.** When they are around four or five years old, give them tools to use such as "Stop, take five, and think" and "Keep your hands and feet to your-

self." One mom says she interferes only when someone is getting hurt; this way it doesn't look like she's taking sides.

- **Put a lid on tattletales.** Yes, it's often enlightening when one twin rats the other out. However, encouraging this dynamic could lead to more trouble than it's preventing. One twin may think she is elevating her position with you while putting her twin in a bad light. If one twin consistently squeals, try not to praise or reward her for the info.

TLC FOR SOTS (SIBLINGS OF TWINS)

Almost half of our survey moms have at least one child in addition to the twins. If your multiples have older or younger siblings, you *can* nurture a healthy dynamic so that no one feels excluded. Of course, your kids' individual and group behavior will vary depending on whether they are tired, hungry, sick, bored, and more. Sometimes the twins will make your singleton feel like the odd one out, but their alliances will shift depending on what they want from each other and what kind of a reaction they get from you. Ages, stages, and gender also play roles in how they all get along. Some moms have singletons who are eighteen months (or less) older or younger than their twins—which means they are often mistaken for triplets. Having a sound routine for the twins that incorporates the schedules and needs of your other kids will help reduce the unpredictability that kids naturally throw your way. Other tips to help all of your kids feel included and special:

- **Rely on your wing man.** Forty percent of the moms in our survey said one of the best things Dad can do when the twins are born is taking care of the other kids. Or Dad can do twin duty so Mom can bond with the singleton(s).
- **Mix and match.** Since convenience often dictates that you treat the twins as a unit and the single sibling(s) as another, it may help foster bonds between all of your kids to occasionally break up the twins and pair one and then the other with the singleton(s). If there is an odd man out, capitalize on the one-on-one time.
- **Create family-wide fun.** Facilitate bonding experiences for everyone to enjoy together (Friday game nights, a Sunday afternoon tee-ball game, or silly story time in the middle of the week).

Extra-Special Twin Families

In our minds, every family with a set of twins is special. We talked to moms who've adopted twins or relied on surrogacy to have their twins to discover how they handle some sensitive subjects and strengthen their family bond.

- They've prepared pat answers for well-intentioned questions such as "Who was born first?" "How was the pregnancy?" or "How many minutes apart were they?"
- They've released the news on a need-to-know basis. The twins are often told from an early age about how they became a family, and it is told as a very positive, happy story. One mom reads her twins the children's book *Tell Me About the Day I Was Born*, by Jamie Lee Curtis. Doctors, teachers, and caregivers are also told up front.
- They've reassured their other kids, whether adopted or biological, that they are all *real* siblings, even if they are not related by blood.

12

DOUBLES' DEVELOPMENT

As a parent of twins, you will inevitably find yourself comparing their emotional, verbal, physical, social, or intellectual development, at least in your thoughts. And that's not necessarily a bad thing. "In the case of developmental milestones, comparison can be useful," says Daddy Doc. "If one twin is lagging significantly behind his sibling, that discrepancy can be a cause for concern and should be brought to the attention of your twin's pediatrician. In particular, identical twins tend to develop more similarly. Any large variation in their developmental course can be a concern."

ACKNOWLEDGING DEVELOPMENTAL DIFFERENCES

Sometimes twins operate at their own pace, particularly if one has medical issues, a common cause of developmental differences. About 10 percent of the survey moms said they experienced pronounced discrepancies in how their twins developed.

Of these moms, most said the differences were either physical or emotional, while some said they were verbal. Once you acknowledge that your twins do things at different paces, what do you do next?

Hit the books. It's helpful to have a reference book or Web site that takes you month by month or year by year through the developmental milestones of a young child. Many survey moms suggested *Babytalk* magazine, babycenter.com, and *The Baby Book* by William Sears, M.D., and Martha Sears, R.N. (Little, Brown, 1993). If you know what is generally expected of your child as an individual—not in relation to his or her twin—you can use that information to guide your decision making when it comes to helping *each* of your twins reach milestones or assessing their progress. Our survey moms of preemies tell us that they have to factor in their babies' adjusted age (their current chronological age minus the number of weeks they were born early) when measuring developmental milestones. This can go on for up to two or three years. Daddy Doc adds, "While twins tend to develop at slower rates than singletons, those delays are more a function of prematurity than twinship."

Keep track of their physical growth. Anytime you get your twins weighed and measured, jot down the results before you forget them. It's interesting to see if one is consistently bigger than the other, or if they do a switcheroo at some point. Don't be discouraged if your twins seem to be smaller than other kids their age—it could just be a twin thing. Daddy Doc says that several studies have looked into twin growth throughout childhood. "They have consistently found that twins have slightly lower BMIs (body mass indexes) and are slightly shorter than their target predicted height when compared to singletons."

Daddy Doc: Understanding Twins and Language Development

Studies show that twins are slower than age-matched singletons when it comes to language development, even when controlled for prematurity. Boy/boy twins are the most delayed, while girl/girl twins develop faster. (Boy/girl twins are in the middle.) According to Daddy Doc, this relative delay is most pronounced between one and two years old. Why the delays? He says that twins tend to reinforce their own immature speech patterns, commonly called twin-speak. "This lingering type of babbling delays the emergence of real language, but not significantly," says Daddy Doc. "Most twins between one and two years will have some secret language, but as long as they also understand whatever their native language is and are progressing with their language development, it is not cause for concern.

"The other reason twins tend to be slightly language-delayed is that they have fewer quality language interactions with family. We all hate to admit it, but twins do get less attention than they would if they were singletons. Parents are stressed, pulled in many different directions simultaneously, and thus we have less time to talk or read to our twins. This lack of parental attention does contribute to slower emergence of speech. The good news about twin language development is that even though they are slower to talk, twins do not suffer permanent delays. The vast majority of twins approach normal by the time they are two or two and a half years old."

Boost twins' egos. One mom says she constantly reassures her twins and lets them know that each person is unique in their own way and has their own special talents to share with others and that some people are better at different things than others.

Be patient. Cathy's fraternal boys did everything at their own pace in the first eighteen months. One was consistently months ahead of the other in walking, talking, and reasoning. But Cathy had enough mommy experience with her two older boys and their peers to know that her slower-paced twin would eventually catch up and develop his own strengths along the way. Plus, she regularly touched base with the twins' pediatrician to keep her concerns in check. She also saw the twin relationship as advantageous, as the more eager twin would gently prod the more relaxed twin to keep up with him, especially when it came to crawling, cruising, walking, and running.

Seek professional help. In more serious cases, some moms said that they've been proactive in seeking out an occupational, physical and/or speech therapist who makes house calls, with continued support in preschool and kindergarten.

Twins Versus Singletons

We wondered what our moms thought about parenting their twins through different milestones and transitions versus what they thought it was like for the parents of singletons they know. Here's how our respondents rated the following:

- Switching from nursing to bottles—almost 60 percent said about the same as singletons
- Giving up bottles—60 percent said about the same as singletons
- Moving from cribs to beds—44 percent said about the same as singletons
- Getting the kids to talk—44 percent said about the same as singletons
- Potty training—35 percent said about the same as singletons
- Getting children adjusted to school—46 percent said about the same as singletons and 20 percent said somewhat easier

If you are still deep in the double diaper trenches, the day you send your twins to kindergarten may seem light-years away. But trust us, it's not. Before the school bus pulls up in front of your house, you have a homework assignment from the Twin Set Moms: find out what your state's policy is on whether or not parents of multiples can choose to have their twins in the same classroom.

"Some teachers and school systems believe that twins need to be separated for their own good," says Daddy Doc. "Yet several studies call that belief into question." To date, Minnesota, Texas, and Georgia are the only states that have legally given parents of multiples this authority. Eight other states, including Pennsylvania and New York, have introduced similar legislation.

A mom from our very own Moms of Multiples club is lobbying state legislators in Connecticut. Her advice: "If someone is interested in starting their own state petition, they should contact twinslaw.com. It's an unbelievable resource. There's so much information on the Internet today, there's just *no* excuse for parents with preschool-age children not to be well informed. If you believe your children may benefit from staying together, get your information together, and speak with your pediatrician, therapists, and counselors. Also, consider hiring a private advocate in your area who is familiar with the school, administrators, and policies. These people will undoubtedly pay for themselves in outcome and peace of mind."

For the latest updates, you can also check out twinsmagazine.com.

Twincidentals: When Preemie Twins Need Separate

Schools Most of the moms who took our survey emphasized the importance of being fair with their twins and seeing them as unique individuals, yet in the context of preemie parenting, it's about recognizing that each twin may have different health and developmental issues. In some cases, this might mean that they go to different preschools or kindergartens, which is not something most parents of twins would consider under other circumstances. The moms we talked to were very reassuring that the twin bond continues when they are back at home, after the school day is over.

Depending on what kind of twins you have, how clingy they are, or how on target they are developmentally, deciding whether to separate them in preschool, kindergarten, or beyond may be a tough call for you (and educators) to make. We're the first generation to face these issues in such vast numbers, so school administrations and boards need to learn about the pros and cons of twin separation from us. Here's some food for thought.

Together

Pros: *Twins are accustomed to spending time together, and this may ease the transition to kindergarten. They may be so different already that they will naturally gravitate toward their own friends and activities without hampering the other, yet they have the comfort of the other twin nearby if need be.*

Cons: They may distract each other from learning or developing new friends and reaching their individual potential. One may protect the other too much and keep him or her from learning how to speak up for him or herself.

Tips: Research potential schools' twin separation policies in advance. In Cathy and Christina's town, for example, some preschools prefer separation, while others are more willing to work with the parents' requests. If you are going to keep your twins together, establish contact with their teacher before Day One and keep that communication channel open all year. Empower the teacher with ways to distinguish the twins with details of their personalities and what each needs to work on. Encourage him or her to seat them at different tables and occupy them at different activities. Consider what grade your twins are going to enter and what they will face academically. It may be trickier for twins to separate in first grade than kindergarten, for example, because things tend to get more challenging for kids academically, and adding the trauma of twin separation to the workload may be too much.

Apart

Pros: *If they are very similar and attached, this might give them their first chance to spread their wings. If one twin is more extroverted, the more introverted one might be more compelled to try new things without his or her twin there. They may also get along better at home if they are not together all day at school.*

Cons: Your twins may miss each other dearly and feel extreme discomfort in the classroom without their support system by their side. Your twins may be so used to going together to Mommy and Me classes or preschool that learning independently, outside that dual environment, may be a shock.

Tips: Talk to their teachers about facilitating twin time during lunch and recess. If your twins are anxious at first, encourage them to sit together at lunch or on the bus. After they get the hang of school, they may be more inclined to sit with their own friends and sporadically—and organically—check in with each other during the school day. If your twins are having a tough time with separation and showing signs of anxiety or depression (loss of appetite, change in sleep patterns, unwillingness to go to school) get the school psychologist on board for an evaluation—you may have to rethink your decision.

TWINS' SOCIAL DEVELOPMENT

Your twins may be particularly adept at making friends in school settings. Daddy Doc says that research from several studies indicates that twins in school settings are more prosocial than their singleton peers. It seems pretty obvious to parents of twins that the advantage comes from the twin-specific environment: you have to learn how to get along with a peer if she is living with you, sleeping with you, and always doing the same things you are. In our survey, the majority of moms agreed that it's easier to have twins adjust to going to school than their singleton peers. However, some twins are shy, and some play date or party invitations can give you a headache. Here are some solutions to sticky twin social situations.

Twincidentals: Ready to Launch When your twins are small and their personalities are still revealing themselves day after day, it's exciting to imagine what they will be like when they are a little older and ready for school. The anticipation of seeing them engage in social settings is both fun and nerve-racking. Will they both be interested in doing the same things? Will they have the same friends? Will one be more social than the other? Will they find friends who understand them more than they do each other? It's hard to stand back and observe, but the way your twins behave when they are out in the big world is special to witness.

Problem: *"Only one of my twins was invited to a birthday party."*
Solution: Not everyone knows how to navigate twin etiquette issues. Other parents may even think it's better to invite *neither* of your children than to risk hurting one twin's feelings. Twenty-five percent of survey moms said that one of their twins has missed out on being invited to a play date or a party because he or she has a twin. Here are some suggestions for handling a situation where only one twin is invited:

1. Let one twin go to the party and set up a play date or do something special with the one at home. You may need to remind the twins that they are different people with different friends, to nip any teasing or competitiveness in the bud.
2. RSVP and ask if it's okay if your other twin joins the fun as well. This may make your life better as a mom of twins, but some hostesses may consider it a brazen move.
3. Keep both twins home, to avoid hurting one's feelings. Just pray that the other doesn't find out he or she is missing a party.
4. Consider that by kindergarten, there tend to be more gender-specific parties, so this problem might become less of an issue if you have boy/girl twins.

Problem: *"People don't realize my twins are twins."*
Solution: Be prepared for the fact that your twins will outgrow the double stroller, not want to wear similar outfits, and may end up in separate classrooms. It might feel new and shocking for you not to get that immediate twin recognition. Our friends with older twins have told us that when their twins entered kindergarten and were in separate classrooms, some of their friends and their friends' parents didn't know they were twins. You can take charge and e-mail the parents in your twins' class(es) about your attitude toward play dates and parties (the twins are a package deal, or individual invites are fine). Or you can hang back and take each situation as it comes.

Twincidentals: When Twins Get Labeled Sometimes

acquaintances may react to what they quickly observe on the surface and assign labels like "the shy one" or "the handful." These reactions may bother you: 47 percent of our survey respondents said they wished their friends and the parents of their twins' friends knew it was bad to compare the twins to each other. When Christina's boy/girl twins are called something in comparison to each other, especially when it is behavior-based, she's quick to defuse the comment by responding, "Well, we all have our moments and every day with these characters is different." It's her way of saying that what you see right now is not entirely accurate or indicative of their true charm or behavioral patterns.

Problem: *"Both my twins get invited to play with this one child, but only one of the twins really likes him."*

Solution: Just send over the twin who actually enjoys being on the play date, saying that the other one can't make it. Try to keep the other twin busy at home or out doing something special. If you have this child over to your house, make sure the twin who doesn't click with him knows you expect her to be nice—but that doesn't mean she has to play with him. You can help her keep busy with a special project while her twin plays with the friend. Don't rule out the possibility that the twins will change their opinion of this friend. They might end up switching their positions, so keep the friend's mom updated.

13

. . . .

GOOD HEALTH

. . . .

*f*or moms of twins, one of the most important things you can do for your children is to promote their good health. That might mean comforting both twins and helping them to be brave while one gets a shot and the other cries in anticipation or sympathy, soothing sick twins in the doctor's waiting room when their desired remedy is to be in your arms, or helping nervous twins relax on their first trip to the dentist. These are often the times when both twins need you at once and you will find yourself—very quickly and instinctively—performing the necessary triage in your mind: who gets Mom first?

It helps to prepare for these difficult days and to take steps to minimize the burden on you and your children. When it comes to the health of your twins, being proactive, knowledgeable, and attentive is the best course of action.

Putting healthy routines in place and being proactive in managing your twins' health care is one of your top priorities as a parent, and establishing a healthy relationship with your children's doctor is step number one. Finding a pediatrician who understands twin-related issues and is comfortable treating your children in relation to each other is very important. You look to your doctor for advice on everything, from how and when to feed your babies to how to treat all kinds of illnesses and ailments, from asthma to the stomach flu. New babies see their doctors quite frequently, for both well and sick visits.

The truth is, a supportive pediatrician can make a difference from the start. Many survey mothers told us they were able to breast-feed their twins thanks to their pediatricians who cheered them on, let them borrow their scales, and persistently reminded them what a great gift they were giving their babies. By the same token, many women told us they felt less horrific switching to formula bottles after getting the nod from their twins' doctors (sans guilt trip). In many ways, your twins' doctor takes care of you as a mom, too, so make sure you're comfortable with his or her approach toward you as well as your twins.

Our Mommy and Daddy Docs offer great insight because their advice to patients is rigorously tested with their own twins day after day. Our Mommy Doc says: "I think for basic medical care, pediatricians without 'twin knowledge' can do a great job. When it comes to many issues related to the twin relationship, I think a pediatrician with that knowledge would have a lot more to add to the conversation. Topics that come to mind are potty-training two at the same time, birthday party dilemmas, sleep survival with two infants, and whether or not to separate in school."

And Daddy Doc weighs in: "It is important for parents to find physicians they feel comfortable talking to. All pediatricians care for some twins in their practice, but there are differences in style and acceptance. Some doctors 'get it' that twins are different and have developmental, psychological, and physical challenges that singletons do not face. Since my own twin girls were born, the biggest difference I have found in dealing with my twin parents is that I can better relate to their struggles. Raising twins can be very difficult and poses physical, emotional, and psychological challenges that are different from singletons, and even different from siblings close in age."

HOW TO EVALUATE A PEDIATRIC PRACTICE OR GROUP

We are confident that many qualified and loving doctors could fulfill your twins' needs. During your search, evaluate potential doctors and practices in light of some twin-friendly characteristics and habits:

- **They offer variety.** Do you need one point of contact or are you comfortable seeing a whole office? The pros of working with a pediatric group include access to several points of view: an old-school approach or more progressive thinking, males and females, young and old, those who treat aggressively or are more "wait-and-see" types. Difficulties can arise when you get out of sync with one or more of the doctors—when they do see your children, they are not quite connected or familiar with them other than via their charts. To find a nice balance, book appointments with your preferred doctor(s) for well visits, and save your flexibility for sick visits when you might be more willing to see anyone who can help.
- **They accept your insurance.** Babies, even those born at full term with no serious health issues, visit the doctor a lot. Despite having

access to great insurance plans, we have both been surprised at the amount of out-of-pocket expenses we accrue with our twins: office visit co-pays, prescription co-pays, over-the-counter products, and so on. We suggest thinking long and hard before deciding to select a pediatrician who is out of your network or plan coverage, where costs can grow very quickly.

- **They will see Mom and Dad, too.** It could be most efficient for you and your family to consider a family medical practice, where one office sees your whole family.

- **They are flexible in scheduling appointments.** For parents of twins, flexibility and a willingness to accommodate your family's special circumstances are important. For example, there are times when one of your twins will be sick in the morning, you'll make an afternoon appointment and by the time it rolls around, your other twin will be showing signs of illness, too. Will your doctor—or others in the office—give you a hassle when you show up with two patients? Certainly you will pay for the second visit as well, but some offices might frown upon a twin crashing his or her twin's time slot.

- **They are easy to communicate with.** What is the office's protocol for calling in with questions or handling crises? Will you get lost in voice mail oblivion? As mothers of multiple toddlers, you can pretty much count on facing some emergency situations. Will your doctors be able to meet your needs?

- **They are convenient.** On the most practical of levels, consider these points: Is the office accessible? Can you fit your double stroller through the doorway? Are stairs involved? What's the parking situation? Carrying two kids across a busy street in the rain to get to the doctor's office is not an ideal situation. Nor is heading out to the car, crying toddlers in tow, via a dark and scary parking garage. Also, the closer the doctor's office to your home or office, the better. In terms of accessibility, don't forget to look into what kind of hours the office keeps. Do they have early morning walk-in hours? Does their voice mail kick in after 4:30 P.M.? Do they have weekend hours? Do they take an hour-long lunch break?

When Both Parents Work

We know from personal experience that the delicate balance maintained by working parents can get whacked out when, for example, you have a vital presentation to deliver at work *and* one or more of your children come down with something. When you literally can't be in two places at the same time, communicating with your twins' physician is crucial. Our Mommy and Daddy Docs have some pointers to help things go smoothly, enhanced by their perspectives as working parents.

Mommy Doc says, "Sending a note in to the doctor's office with the specific symptoms and questions is very helpful. A lot of times the child care provider can't answer questions about symptoms that occur at night or over the weekend because he or she hasn't been with the children. Also, a parent leaving a phone number and being available via phone at the time of the visit is helpful. This way, the doctor can call to explain the diagnosis and the plan. It is very important that a working mom find a doctor who is willing to take that extra minute to call and communicate with her."

Daddy Doc concurs, saying: "Physicians have had to change our practice styles to meet the needs of working families. We have expanded office hours, and most groups have early morning hours, evening hours, or both. Parents can help by making sure that the caretaker they entrust their children to is knowledgeable about the health situation. When I examine a child, it's important for me to know specifics about the illness: how long the cough has been going on, whether it is worse at night or all day long, what the throw-up looks like, whether the rash is itchy or not, etc. I communicate with working parents via cell phone and e-mail while their children and caretaker are still in the office. While it has definite limitations, I advise my families to e-mail me for non-urgent questions or things they just want to run past me but don't need a visit for."

When Mommy Knows Best

Doctors provide information, advice and care, but the parental vantage point is a powerful tool, too. It's telling that barely 7 percent of the moms we surveyed said they get their best twin-specific parenting advice from their doctors/pediatricians. Instead, they rely heavily on Mothers of Multiples clubs and other friends for advice and guidance. And when that network is absent or lacking in advice, you'll learn to rely on your own maternal instinct. It might not be easy to listen to your gut, given your personal lack of medical training. But the truth is, no one knows your twins better than you do. Most doctors see many patients each day, encompassing a variety of ailments and at a variety of ages and stages. The doctor who diagnosed your child's ear infection one day might not necessarily be the one doing the recheck a week later. As parents, we have access to the whole picture, so it's up to us to fill in the blanks and provide the gut check when necessary.

BREAKING UP IS HARD TO DO

There might come a time when you realize that your pediatric practice just doesn't seem to get your twins' needs. You've probably been through some emotional bonding with your children's pediatrician. But if something is not right, it's time to start looking around. Leaving a practice does not mean the doctors are not competent or caring; it might simply mean that you have some special twin needs that might be better served elsewhere. Here are some tips to help you find a new practice.

- **Define your issues and where the current practice is lacking** so you'll know, and be able to articulate, what you're looking for.
- **Ask for referrals from friends and other parents of twins.** Again, ask pointed questions of them so you really understand what it is your friend likes about her twins' doctor.
- **Ask for a meeting with the doctor(s).** Conduct the discussion much like a job interview. This is your first glimpse into whether or

not they are willing to entertain your questions and concerns. And be prepared: when you start looking around, you may conclude that your current doctor is not so bad after all.

Write down your questions and discussion topics beforehand. A lot can distract you from your time with the doctor, so it helps to go through your checklist during the visit. Cathy writes her list for each child in her planner on the page for the day of the scheduled well-child visit, since at her pediatrician's office appointments for these checkups are made roughly three months in advance.

Bring your double stroller as long as possible. Even if you have begun ditching your stroller for other outings, it can come in handy at the doctor's office. If your twins are sick, you won't want them crawling around the office getting everyone else sick. If they aren't sick, you won't want them running about touching all the germy surfaces. Don't forget your tools. It helps to

When Twins Need Medical Specialists

Sometimes one or both of your twins will require the care of a specialist. Babies born prematurely, in particular, tend to need follow-up care from pulmonologists, physical therapists, or ophthalmologists. Typically, your pediatrician can provide recommendations. Again, the most important criterion in selecting a doctor is his or her sensitivity to your twins' needs and your challenges as their parent—although with specialists, the extent of their twin-specific experience might be limited.

have a stocked bag: something to bribe/reward good behavior, water or something else for them to drink, diapers and wipes, and something to comfort them for shots. It also helps to bring antibacterial wipes or hand sanitizer with you.

Put your game face on. If your twins are sick, the visit can take an emotional toll on you, too. It's hard to see someone stick a long swab down your child's throat for a culture. Even if the kids are well, they might need shots, and it is tough to comfort them after you just aided and abetted the nurse by holding them down. Sometimes you'll need to ask the doctor difficult or complex questions, all the while managing the logistics and your lists. Try to remain calm so your children can follow your cues. Or consider bringing Dad, Grandma, or a sitter to help.

MANAGING THE PAPERWORK

If you have health insurance, you'll need to spend a good deal of time dealing with all of the paperwork. Here are some suggestions for streamlining the process.

To Bring or Not to Bring

Fifty-seven percent of the moms we surveyed said they sometimes take the seemingly healthy twin to the doctor with the sick twin, 9 percent said they always bring both, and 34 percent never bring a healthy twin to the doctor. Bringing both twins can mean extra TLC for the sick twin who is getting poked and prodded. Or it can mean the well twin, jealous of the attention the sick one is receiving, will start acting out. Whenever possible, we try to leave healthy kids at home with Dad or a sitter or a friend. Why expose them to all the germs in the waiting room if we can avoid it?

Consider the co-pays. It's tempting to bring along a semi-sick twin to get checked out when a really sick twin needs to be examined by the doctor. But that's a minimum of $20 in co-pays out of your pocket each time, so don't take it lightly. The costs associated with health care might require that you be more selective in terms of when and how often your twins are reviewed by the doctor. Of course, nothing should stand in the way of your children's good health, but considering your budget might be a good idea.

Flex your money muscles. Flexible spending accounts (FSAs) are great because they allow you to put pre-tax dollars aside for medical expenses not covered by insurance. If you don't use all the money you set aside over the course of a year, however, you lose it. Learning how to budget the right amount is important. Get in the habit of saving your receipts for over-the-counter essentials for sick twins, such as Tylenol or Motrin—you can use a flex spending account for all of these expenses. You can also use it for prescription co-pays and medical expenses not covered by your insurance. By keeping all of your prescription and over-the-counter receipts in one place and tallying up costs quarterly, you can see how much of a balance remains and start thinking about your FSA target for the following year.

Manage multiple prescriptions. Some insurance plans provide discounts on regularly used prescription medications if you order them in advance and receive them through the mail. This might save a busy mom of twins several trips to the pharmacy. Keeping prescriptions straight is another twin-related challenge. Two children with the same birthday, same last name, and maybe adorable twin-matching first names could mean confusion when it comes to medical charts, insurance paperwork, and even phoned-in prescriptions. Be vigilant and try to use full first names (and middle names if you have to) in all dealings.

TWO OUNCES OF PREVENTION

It is nearly impossible to keep twins from sharing their germs, but there are some easy steps you can take to minimize the impact of one twin's illness on the other. Daddy Doc says: "Twins share everything. Bottles, pacifiers, toys—every object that one of my daughters has will inevitably wind up in the hands of the other

Twin Set Confidential: Shh! Our Twins Have Shared Prescription Medicine

It's natural that your twins will come down with the same illness a few days apart. If you've already dragged one to the doctor at the beginning of the week, it's not appealing to drag the other there a couple of days later when you are pretty sure the diagnosis is going to be the same. A mom of twins may be tempted to use one twin's prescription medication on the other. Christina has done it, and so has Cathy. Once or twice, when Cathy's twins were sick with terrible colds and being treated for breathing issues, she filled a prescription and ended up using half of the doses for the prescribed child and the other half for his twin.

That behavior, while helpful when you just want your children to breathe freely, does have consequences. Splitting the dosage means you run out twice as fast as your insurance company expects you to, so you might have trouble refilling a prescription for the original child. Your doctor can help you deal with this, but you might get reprimanded in the process.

sooner or later. This naturally leads to the spread of germs throughout homes with twins. Families always share germs, but with two or more infants or toddlers, it can be very hard to control. I recommend a few steps to stay on top of the massive germ onslaught. Keeping up to date on the recommended vaccines, including flu shots, gives your twins a leg up. Keeping germs out of the house also goes a long way. Several good studies have found that families that used antibacterial hand sanitizers liberally during illnesses had significantly lower rates of spread within the household."

Mommy Doc adds, "Just washing hands is the best means of preventing the sharing of germs." Other options: labeling bottles or cups, assigning each twin a color for cups and bottles, and using individual medicine dispensers and medical supplies for each twin. To avoid confusing one twin's prescription with the other's, consider using the pharmacy at your local Target, which can use different-colored-rings on prescription bottles for different family members.

LIFE WITH SICK TWINS

It's amazing how much havoc a simple cold can wreak in a twin household. Personally, we've been knocked down from our type A personality perches when both of our twins are sick. Other times it's not so bad. One mother told us her twins naturally seemed to split their illnesses, so one is healthy when the other is sick. And, she added, the well one tends to be sympathetic to the sick one and allow him or her to get the special attention needed from Dr. Mom without jealousy or fighting. That hasn't happened in our homes, but we hope your twins will be well behaved and understanding when one of them is sick!

We wondered if there were common ailments that tend to occur more frequently in twins, but according to both Mommy Doc and Daddy Doc, there is not much existing medical research out there related to twin children. The most common health issues they encounter with their twin patients are a result of prematurity. Mommy Doc adds some insight: "Theoretically, any disease that has a genetic component to it would have an increased incidence in identical twins. Asthma, allergies, and autoimmune disorders are some examples."

Here are some insights and tips for dealing with some of the regular childhood ailments happening in double time.

Colic. Cathy's second son (a singleton) was described by his pediatrician as colicky, so she feels somewhat qualified to describe the symptoms: inconsolable crying fits that can occur daily for weeks or months. It might be limited to the evening hours or, as in the case of Cathy's son, last throughout the day and night (seriously). Daddy Doc adds, "Colic, which is a descriptive term, is *very* frustrating for parents. We need to see those babies to make sure nothing else is wrong. But if they are growing well and have a normal physical exam, parents can be comforted by knowing that their baby will outgrow the fussiness." Colic is very difficult to deal with because no matter what you do, you can't seem to provide comfort to your child. Plus, the constant screaming is difficult on the nerves. Even if only one of your babies seems to be colicky, you're still not having an easy time of it. The good news is: the day it's over, it's over. Some describe it as a switch turning off, and for Cathy's son, that is exactly what it was like. The bad news is that it can be a long waiting period. Daddy Doc sympathizes: "Colic tends to get worse at about four to six weeks and then improve at about six months. The only remedy that definitely works is time."

Reflux. Mommy Doc says that twins tend to have reflux because of prematurity. So what is reflux? It stems from an immature esophageal sphincter, which normally prevents the stomach contents from coming back up the esophagus. Daddy Doc adds, "All babies spit up, but some *really* spit up all the time. Sometimes that can be a marker for serious medical conditions, so let your pediatrician know about it. If your baby is gaining weight well, then it is probably reflux. Sometimes we order ultrasounds or swallowing studies to make sure. The first thing to try is changing a nursing mother's diet or switching formulas. These dietary changes work for some babies, but to be honest, it is frequently more frustrating than helpful for parents to change formulas or the mother's diet. Sometimes your baby's physician will recommend medicine such as Zantac, Axid, or other antacids. These work for some babies. Most babies with reflux will outgrow it between six and twelve months. But those can be *very long* months."

Thrival Tip: The Tiny Miracles Foundation's Web site, ttmf.org, is a wonderful resource, recommended by our Mommy Doc, with links to many organizations that can help educate parents about illnesses related to premature birth.

Twin Sets of Teeth

Most children begin visiting the dentist at age three. For twins, the mob mentality can impact the event. On the positive side, if the first patient is excited and enjoys the special attention and token prize and toothbrush, it can serve to allay any fears the second might have. On the other hand, one bad reaction and suddenly nobody wants to go near the dentist's chair. If you think they will both freak out, maybe try to take one at a time (many dentists offer Saturday hours, so you and Dad can tag-team). For Christina, both three-year-old twins seemed scared during their first visit. She sat in the examination chair with her crying daughter on her lap. After some persuasion, her daughter finally relaxed and let the dentist count her teeth and clean them. But her son would barely even sit in the examination chair with her. He refused to open his mouth for the counting part. For the next visit, six months later, both twins were much more relaxed and sat in the examination chair by themselves. Her son had a full counting and cleaning. What a difference half a year makes!

Teething. While not an ailment, teething is painful for your twins. There is definitely crying involved, and it can affect sleeping and eating habits, too. When twins share a room and one or both are up screaming because of teething in the middle of the night, there are limited things you can do for their pain management. We've offered the suffering twin everything from Tylenol to ice pops to cold, wet washcloths for comfort. Seventy-five percent of the moms we surveyed said they treat this condition on an individual basis; pain meds for one does not dictate pain meds for the other one.

Terrific Twinsight: One of our moms with identical twins had her dentist tell her the twins had almost identical teeth. Pretty cool.

Ear infections. A lot of children suffer ear infections, especially between twelve and twenty-four months. This is a time when kids tend to battle cold after cold and suffer through every virus that comes within a five-mile radius. Cathy's first two singleton sons had a few ear infections each, but nothing out of the ordinary. Her twins, on the other hand, seemed to suffer from double ear infections with every common cold. The doctor told her it was a simple issue of anatomy: their ears were not draining properly. They each underwent surgery to have tubes implanted within six weeks of each other. The ordeal of the surgeries was tough on Cathy and her husband, but her guys went from antibiotic after antibiotic to good health right away. One son's overall disposition improved, too, and she assumes it was because he had been in constant discomfort from the fluid in his ears.

Stomach illnesses. When they are vomiting at the same time, you need to act quickly and decisively: contain one and begin to clean up the other. When tummy traumas reach Category Five level, the best you can do is comfort and pursue a policy of containment. Start by noticing cues early on: if one of your twins isn't eating well while the other is sick, it's probably a heads-up that your other twin might be coming down with it, too. One mom we know strips her kids down to diapers and/or undies when they have the pukes or the runs. She also strips the beds down to just fitted sheets on top of plastic mattress covers, and then places the mattresses on the floor next to her bed. This makes middle-of-the-night sickness easier to clean up.

Asthma/lung congestion. Many children today are treated for asthma-related illnesses. Even common colds can escalate and lead to the need for steroid medication administered directly into the lungs through a machine called a nebulizer. Both Cathy and Christina have used these machines to administer two kinds of liquid medicine to their twins. The tricky part is holding a mask over a toddler's face so she can breathe in the medication (it can take about ten minutes) while keeping her twin from unplugging the machine or playing with the on/off button. The trickier part is having to nebulize both twins several times a day for a few days. We cut down the nebulizer time by literally combining the two medications into one breathing treatment (our doctors' idea). Depending on how often your twins need to be nebulized, you might want to consider renting or buying two machines so they can be treated simultaneously. Also, it's important to have individual masks or mouthpieces for each twin. We store these in labeled plastic bags or containers to keep them straight.

Twincidentals: Sick for Attention

Now that Christina's twins are older, they aren't always sick at the same time anymore, even though they share a room. That said, when one is sick, the other will often pretend to be sick, too, to get attention. Sometimes the well twin will get upset when Christina gives the sick twin medicine. The well twin will carry on even though Christina tries to explain that he is lucky not to be sick. The sick twin will rub it in—"Ha ha, I get to take medicine," even if it tastes yucky and she just gave Christina a hard time about swallowing it. Christina has filled a medicine dropper with fake "medicine" before (water mixed with food coloring) and given it to the well twin, just to keep things peaceful. And we've all put Band-Aids on invisible boo-boos, right?

TIPS FOR SURVIVING BEING HOUSEBOUND
AND SLEEP-DEPRIVED (AGAIN)

Sick twins are usually not themselves because they aren't eating or sleeping well, which translates into Mom and Dad not eating or sleeping well. It's understandable that parents might run out of patience with whining twin patients—and with each other. Before your family has a group meltdown, try taking the ick out of sick.

- **Find a drugstore that delivers or has drive-through service.** If you think it's hard to unbuckle and carry in two healthy twins, try two sick twins!
- **Get over trying to keep your healthy twin from playing with your unhealthy one.** You can do your best to keep them from sharing toys, but you'll soon see that your efforts are pretty much futile (at least our efforts always were). Clean their stuff as well as possible when they are down at night. Lysol spray and wipes rule!
- **Keep a supply of stomach-related remedies at home.** Load up on Pedialyte or Gatorade, FeverAll (a fever reducer that is administered rectally when children are vomiting), and tummy-friendly foods such as saltine crackers, white rice, and applesauce. The last thing you want to do is strap two vomiting kids into their car seats and head to the store for these supplies.
- **Record which twin took what medication and when.** It's stressful to remember details when you are exhausted. Write it down or use a digital tool such as the Itzbeen (also mentioned in our "Chow Time" and "Pee and Poop" chapters), a device that helps parents remember the baby care details.

Medicate yourself, too. No, we're not suggesting mother's little helper here. Rather, acknowledge the mental and emotional toll caring for two sick children can take on you. Oftentimes when children are sick only Mommy will do. We generally feel like we have things relatively under control, but when one or both of our twins are sick, all bets are off. Suddenly you're living the "Calgon, take me away" commercial from years ago. Everyone's in pajamas, no one sets foot outside the house, and dishes and laundry pile high. Your only focus becomes tending to the sick, and your personal well-being falls to the bottom of the list. We encourage you to work in some stress reducers: ask for help from your husband, parents, neighbors, or babysitter; take a power nap; treat yourself to your favorite chai latte or green tea; take the twins out for a quick walk. Fresh air heals all.

14

SAFETY MATTERS

even the most conscientious parents can't keep their eyes on two active twins at every moment, and as a result, many moms we surveyed found safety and logistics to be the most stressful aspects of raising their twins. Twin-specific safety challenges include one child distracting you from what the other is doing; two children exploring (crawling, walking, then running) in two different directions; two children physically enabling each other to cause trouble or cheering each other on when creating mischief; one child mimicking the other's dangerous behavior (otherwise known as monkey see, monkey do); two tired, sick, or teething children who are more prone to hurting each other; and two children vying for a busy parent's attention and willing to try anything to get it. We try to stay one or two steps ahead of our twins when it comes to their safety, but we're not always successful. Sometimes they outfox, outrun, or outnumber us, and catastrophe strikes.

One of Christina's twins, one of Cathy's twins, and Cathy's middle guy each fell down a full flight of stairs in the same week. Miraculously, none of them was hurt, and they all shook it off rather nicely. Other times, our kids' accidents have had greater consequences, increasing our moments of accident-induced self-doubt. For example, one night Cathy was entertaining her twins when one of them started throwing a fit. They ran in separate directions, one toward a bedroom and one toward the bathroom. She took her eye off the relatively happy one to tend to the screams of the other. In that moment, her happy fellow decided it would be a good time to climb into the bathtub. Luckily, there was no water in it. But he did hit his mouth, fracturing one of his front baby teeth. The gaping hole in his smile will remain that way until his permanent teeth come in (around age six), and reminds Cathy of the gaping hole the accident left in her self-confidence as a parent. But as other parenting successes mute any lingering feelings of failure and guilt, she realizes that both holes will be filled with a little bit of character.

Before you sprout a new white hair, remember that there's only so much you can do to prevent accidents with your twins. That said, here's how to make your home as safe as possible:

Use gates indoors and out. Once twins begin to move, whether crawling or walking, gated play areas are highly recommended by our survey moms to keep them safe and you sane. You can buy sets with add-on sections that allow you to expand it as they get older, creating a nice-size area for two babies to tool around in. The gates from One Step Ahead have activities to distract your twins from climbing over them. Gates or screens are also important for blocking stairs and keeping your twins out of rooms that have not been childproofed.

Stoop to their level. The best way to twinproof your home is to get on your hands and knees and act like your two little mischief makers, searching for sharp corners, electrical outlets, power cords, unsteady lamps, blind cords, fireplaces and heaters, climbing opportunities near windows, toys with small pieces, chemical-filled cabinets, doors that could be shut on little fingers, outer doors that are too easy to open from the inside, and anything that could be toppled on top of them. You can buy solutions to most of the problem areas you discover through the One Step Ahead catalogue, at Home Depot, or in the childproofing section of your local baby store.

Empower yourself. No matter how old your twins are, it's probably a good idea to look into taking a first aid and CPR class. Contact your local Red Cross or adult education facility for more information. Think about having Dad and anyone else who helps care for the twins take these classes as well.

Create a safety zone. It's essential to your sanity to have a room or area of the house where you know the twins can play—sometimes for a few minutes without supervision—without getting hurt or into too much trouble. That means removing or locking away all hazardous and dangerous objects. In Cathy's house, the older boys play in what her husband has dubbed "the varsity playroom" (a converted guest room), where games with little pieces and dice are kept on high shelves, while the toddler twins play in the "JV playroom" (which doubles as the family room and is right off the kitchen), where only toys such as Fisher-Price Little People and wooden puzzles are allowed. All cabinets and drawers are locked or babyproofed in case those toys don't hold the twins' attention.

Terrific Twinsight: "I survived in the beginning with family support and lots of babyproofing."

Cook with caution. Your kitchen may be the most difficult place to keep the twins safe. Cathy has a small kitchen area, and it gets really crowded with three frustrated people in there (two twins who always seem to need to be held right before mealtime and one stressed-out chef/mommy). It's a recipe for danger. We suggest that you separate safe from unsafe utensils and keep the unsafe ones where the twins can't get them, cook only on the back burners of your stove, and either remove or lock your stovetop control dials. Try to be as conscientious as possible about leaving knives, hot pots and pans, and household cleaners within the twins' reach—even if you only intend to set them down for a second. It may help to keep the twins busy when you are cooking, so have toys and art supplies nearby. Some moms cook dinner first thing in the morning, when the twins are still asleep. Remind anyone who comes over to help to follow kitchen safety precautions. And for the times when accidents do happen, keep a first aid kit stashed under the kitchen sink (Johnson & Johnson and 3M make them).

Mind the bathroom. Lots of moms bring their twins in the bathroom with them when they shower. When they are newborns and strapped into bucket car seats, this is an ideal way for moms to relax and enjoy a refreshing break. When they are toddlers, this can become a bit of a mess. Bathrooms are places where your twins can get into a lot of trouble. Risk reducers to consider: installing outside locks on your bathroom doors (so twins can't get in without adult supervision or lock themselves in), never leaving one or both of your twins alone in the tub (they can drown or accidentally or purposely knock each other over and get hurt), making sure your hot water heater isn't set higher than 120 degrees, and hiding medicines, cosmetics, and bathroom cleaners in hard-to-reach or locked cabinets.

Practice fire safety. Every family should have a fire plan, complete with an escape route or two and a meeting place. When your twins are young you should think about how you'd get them out of your home safely if you were there alone with them. Could you carry them both out? Start educating your twins about fire safety as early as possible. You can teach two- and three-year-olds where the fire alarms are in your home and what they sound like; how to get low and call 9-1-1; not to put blankies or clothes on top of lamps; not to touch radiators, heaters, fireplaces, wood-burning stoves, matches, lighters, and candles; and to turn lights off when leaving a room. For more info about family fire safety, talk to your local fire department and check out usfa.gov or sparky.org.

HOW TO GET AROUND YOUR HOME SAFELY WITH YOUR TWINS

Our survey reveals that the number one most stressful thing about being a new mother of twins is figuring out how to physically manage two babies. How you move them and where you put them to play or leave them to wait for you depends on their size and mobility.

The Stairs

Infants in buckets. Take one twin at a time, buckled in the car seat, to the top or bottom of the stairs. Leave babies waiting in buckets in a safe area. Remember that bucket car seats can rock a little bit, so don't leave them close to the top of the stairs.

Babies in your arms. It's tempting to carry the two of them at once, especially if you're rushing or they're both crying for you. Even if you are physically strong, resist the urge to double-scoop. Carrying one twin is safer because you'll have one arm free to help balance yourself or break a fall. Before you hit the stairs, place the waiting baby in a safe zone, such as a portable crib or secured bouncy seat. Put the baby who's just climbed or descended the stairs with you in a safe zone while you retrieve the other baby.

Crawlers. Even though your babies instinctively figured out how to crawl, they're probably going to need help from you to negotiate the stairs. Train one twin at a time, and make sure the twin who's not getting a lesson is in a safe place. To teach crawling down the stairs, you can start at the top of the stairs, get on your hands and knees, and show your baby how to turn around and descend in reverse. Make sure you are in a good position to catch your baby. In between training sessions, keep those safety gates closed at the top and bottom. Once your twins have mastered crawling down the stairs safely (Mommy Doc says probably around fifteen to eighteen months), you may feel comfortable letting both of them on the stairs at the same time. Just be sure to put yourself a couple of steps lower than them, so you are in a position to rescue one or both. Mommy Doc reminds us that even if they seem to have perfected crawling up and down, your twins will still require your supervision for a while.

Toddlers. It takes a while to get the hang of walking up and down the stairs safely. Convincing one stubborn toddler to hold your hand or a stair rail on the way up or downstairs is hard enough. Mommy Doc says that walking upstairs is usually an

Terrific Twinsight: "I wish I knew that it was going to get much easier once the twins were walking. Just getting them from the second floor to the first floor was a logistical nightmare. I'd have to leave one screaming in the crib and run down a flight of stairs to the playroom with the other, whom I would leave screaming in an ExerSaucer. I'd run back up the stairs and get the one in the crib and go back down the stairs. I thought I'd be doing that for the rest of my life."

eighteen-month-old's skill, while walking down is a developmental skill that might not be mastered until the twins are two or three years old. When you can, take the twins for a walk downstairs one at a time, and try to be in a position to catch them. Eventually you can let them walk down the stairs at the same time, emphasizing that they have to hold on (to your hand or the rail), go slow, watch where they are walking, and not push their twin. Mommy Doc recommends that you stick with stair gates until the twins are two or three, and keep them longer if you're concerned about nighttime wandering.

HOW TO KEEP YOUR TWINS SAFE
WHEN YOU'RE OUTSIDE

Fresh air is great for twins and moms alike, but the careful environment you create and control in your home doesn't exactly translate. You need to build a whole new system outdoors. We have always tried to get our twins outside every day for as much time as possible, but it involves constant supervision and a lot of running around. Sometimes the choices you make regarding destination can ease the responsibility. But gates help, too. Here are some general guidelines:

What Makes a Playground Twin-Friendly?

Not all playgrounds are created equal. For a mom with baby twins, a gated, dog-free playground with baby swings in a shaded area is optimal. For a mom with toddler twins, a fenced-in area that's just for kids five and under is ideal. With preschoolers, you can upgrade to a park with big-kid swings and slides. If they act too independent and it's hard for you to see them both, give them boundaries to play within. And if they have trouble following your rules and you are getting stressed out, consider pulling the plug. This way, they'll understand that their behavior has consequences, and you'll get a change of scenery and a chance to cool down.

Do your prep work inside. Put on the gear they'll need (hats, mittens, swim diapers, etc.) before you let them play outside, pop them in the stroller, or load them up in the car to drive to your destination. If they'll need bug spray or sunscreen, you're better off applying those at home, too.

Consider confinement. With twin crawlers, perhaps the most worrisome outdoor culprits are rocks, acorns, small sticks, or anything else they might discover and decide to taste-test. Your twins can still enjoy the benefits of being outside if they are playing on top of a big blanket that's surrounded by a play gate, or if they are in their bouncy seats or ExerSaucers in a shaded area. If you're going to the playground, take your double stroller as long as your twins are still willing to sit in it. (Christina held on to hers until her twins were three.) This takes the stress out of getting the kids from your parked car to the park. It also gives you a place to feed baby twins or put a naughty twin.

When your twins can walk and run, a gated yard can save you a lot of angst. Cathy was able to survive without a gate at the end of her driveway when her two singleton boys were young because their needs were staggered: one was mature enough to follow rules and would reliably stay in the yard just as the other was walking, exploring, and demanding to be chased. Since the twins reached that exploration phase at the same time, the situation became too dangerous for one adult to handle, so the new gates are always closed and locked during their outdoor playtime.

Set strict safety rules. Fencing is expensive and not feasible for many of us. That's where rules come in. Non-negotiable rules include not playing near the street, log pile, creek, or anything that's big and dangerous near where you live. Talk to twins about things they might climb up that they can fall down from. Some twins (like Christina's) may like to bolt in two different directions, and you have to choose which one to grab first. After this happens, you may need to sit them both down and have a chat about listening to Mommy or the other adult in charge if they want to have fun outside. If they can't follow your outdoor rules, it may be time to put them in the stroller and take a walk so you can burn off your frustration and everyone still gets some much-needed fresh air.

Rock-solid safety rules are also essential when you take your twins on a water-related outing: no running on the side of the pool, sitting and waiting on the side of the pool until it's their turn to swim with you, and so on. At the beach, train your twins to approach the water with your permission and with an adult by their side. Praise and reward your twins for following your safety rules.

How Do We Keep Twins Safe?

Relying on confinement methods (such as bouncy seats, baby swings, and play yards) is one of the top three ways survey moms make their day with the twins easier. Almost 20 percent of moms wish their friends with singletons understood that restraint in a stroller is a safety precaution with twins—and it doesn't mean you're a bad mom. Only 7 percent of moms fessed up to using kid leashes with their twins. But we bet many more wish they'd had them at least once!

Water Safety Tips

- **Don't rely on floaties to keep your twins safe.** Inflatable boats and rings with built-in seats can be a mom's lower-back-saver at a kiddie pool. But if your twins lean too far in one direction, these may topple easily. Or other kids in the pool can accidentally tip your twins. That means even with the floaties, you must keep an extra-close eye on them.
- **Stay close.** Your baby twins may prefer to sit on the bottom of the kiddie pool or pull up on the side. Make sure you are within arm's reach so you can pull them up if they fall over (or keep them from drinking the pool water).

Keep a basic first aid kit on hand. If your twins are active, chances are they'll fall and get a few scrapes during your outings. The last thing you want to happen is to have a boo-boo sabotage all the hard work you put into getting everyone out the door and to the playground. A little preparation—Band-Aids and an antibiotic cream in your diaper bag—will go a long way.

Bring help. If your twins have older or younger siblings, you may be faced with a situation that requires you to be in two places at once (the twins want a snack at the concession stand, but their little sister needs a diaper change; the twins are having a blast in the baby pool, but their older brother wants to swim in the big pool). Make outings with your twins and other kids safer and less stressful by bringing a qualified helper. If you are going to economize when it comes to getting extra help, water-related outings are not the area to cut back on.

HOW TO KEEP YOUR TWINS SAFE OUT IN PUBLIC

When they are little and safely strapped into their stroller seats, people fawning over your twins can be the confidence boost a tired mom craves. But when they are a bit older and capable of and/or insistent upon walking by themselves, safety is the paramount concern. Most times, we opted to stick with the stroller, even for short trips across a parking lot for preschool pickup. But other times, you'll want them out and enjoying the environment, such as at an older sibling's soccer game or family picnic. Just realize that you'll need to be constantly vigilant, making it hard to keep score or socialize.

Most moms we talked to say they go for the stroller in as many situations as feasible for as long as possible. Some even joke that the cardinal rule of twin motherhood is never to let them out of the stroller! As an alternative to the stroller, try backpacks. Cathy's twins have been more willing to be mobile on the backs of Mom and Dad rather than strapped in next to their twin.

If they are walking about, try to corral them toward a semi-contained corner of your environment. Set the boundaries right away so they get some sense of where the open space is.

Save your most serious tone of voice and most strident consequences for infractions of the rules out in public. The possibility of a breakaway is always there, but fear can be a powerful deterrent against bad behavior.

15

·············

MONEY

·············

ecent statistics from the Department of Agriculture (the government agency that tracks this data) suggest it will cost somewhere in the neighborhood of $250,000 (geography plays a role in the final number) to raise a child born in 2008 until age eighteen, and upward of $280,000 to send that child to a four-year private college. Parents across America are daily taken aback by such projections—and obviously, as parents of twins, we need to double those figures. Yowch!

Even the most financially savvy people can be caught off guard by the prospect of caring for and raising twins. That's why we're here to let you know what to expect and to share our moms' (and a financial planner's) strategies for making ends meet and saving over time. For parents of twins who've paid for fertility treatments, where multiple births are not an entirely unexpected outcome, there's not as much of an element of surprise at the expenses you'll face. Others, who experience the surprise of a spontaneous twin pregnancy, may be unprepared and perhaps more apprehensive about how they can afford to have two babies.

When Cathy was surprised by the sonogram technician and

learned she was expecting two more babies—in addition to the two young boys she already had—she and her husband went from thinking they could squeeze another car seat into their little station wagon to needing a much bigger vehicle. Other adjustments and purchases were made at the Stahl house: two new cribs (the one they had was occupied and they didn't want to add a forced transition to a bed to the list of anxieties their eighteen-month-old was facing after two baby brothers arrived at once), a double stroller, and more. Rather than feel like parental veterans who had all the equipment and expertise they needed to raise a third baby, Cathy and her husband become scared and overwhelmed "new" parents again. Financially, doubling their number of children had serious repercussions.

One of the distinctions between having multiple children— even those close in age—and having twins is that with twins we're experiencing all of the milestones, phases, and joys at precisely the same time. For John Gugle, a professional financial planner based in Charlotte, North Carolina, and father of fraternal twin boys, the economic hit was no less daunting. He reiterates our collective reaction: "The biggest financial challenge is concurrent expenditures at every step of your child's life—two clothing bills, doctor bills, tuition bills." But, he adds, "any child adds fun and a financial challenge to a family. Twins add more fun and an additional need for financial planning." Seventy-eight percent of the moms we surveyed admit to being surprised by the amount of money they spend on basic necessities for their twins. When it comes to finances, staggering children, even by a year, would be extremely helpful. Luckily, one of the most basic elements of long-term financial security is planning, and that is a skill we parents of twins have been forced to get pretty good at. Now it's time to apply our planning skills to our money mangement: setting goals and budgets, saving and investing over time, and sticking to long-term strategies.

Gugle says the biggest problem is that parents of twins have far less room for financial errors. That's why he says don't wait—start planning as soon as you hear the news that they're coming. The first priority should be to set a budget. Budgeting involves assessing how much you make, how much you spend, and deciding what to do with what's left over. To assess how much of your spending is required and how much is discretionary, ask, "What can we do without?" It might be time to have a discussion with your spouse: Do we need all those cable channels or can we live with basic cable? Do we need an extravagant vacation this year or can we do something locally that's less expensive? Should we cut back on help around the house now, like the lawn mower guy and the snowplow guy, so we can afford help with the twins later? Even if the amount of money you have "left over" for discretionary spending is comfortable for your family, you will be flabbergasted by the amount of money that two little babies can cost. But there are ways to ease the pain. In addition to cutting back on some household expenses, our survey moms shared some general money-saving strategies.

Buy in bulk. This is a great way to maximize savings on things you buy and use for your twins and your home on a regular basis. Most warehouse clubs, such as Costco, Sam's Club, and BJ's, charge an annual membership fee. After that, you can buy large quantities of the stuff you need at a lower per-unit price than the smaller-package options at regular grocery stores and drugstores. At Costco we can buy diapers, ointment, wipes, sippy cups, medicine, formula, and even jars of organic baby food at rates considerably less than local retailers. In addition to the cost savings, buying in bulk saves you from making trips to the store.

Utilize tag sales and twin exchanges. One of the most practical benefits of being a member of a Mothers of Multiples club is access to the exchange of twin equipment. Our local MOMs club hosts an online forum for buying, selling, and donating gently used baby stuff and a semi-annual tag sale where members can buy and sell twin wares. Membership has its privileges! Many of the more expensive items, such as baby swings and portable cribs, are used for such a short time, they are completely viable for resale. Consignment shops are another option.

Thrival Tip: **Saving Money by Keeping Twin Clothes Organized** Clothing your twins is big business. Organizing your twins' clothes can make them accessible and thereby save you from buying new ones, which in turn saves you cash. It takes work to respond to outgrown clothes (toss, save, lend, donate), a change of seasons, and hand-me-downs or gifts. In addition to some common sense, we use big clear plastic storage boxes, cedar blocks and sprays, and labels and Sharpies to organize and put away clothes that don't fit yet, clothes that could be used again in six months, or ones that can be saved for another child.

Another money-saver: the hand-me-down. Sometimes it's hard for moms to accept these gifts because we want our new babies in new clothes, but after weeks and weeks of laundry for two little guys, you might change your tune. Cathy has four boys, so she has become a donation center for used hockey skates, bikes, winter coats, and shoes from all over town. She's even gotten sweaters, shorts, jackets, pants, and shirts from Christina's son, who's just nine months older than her twins. It is all a wonderful help, especially since her little boys seem to ravage clothes and equipment.

Top Five "Out-of-the-Box" Money-Saving Tips Revealed in Our Survey

1. **Utilize free.** Favorites include the park, library, and beach.
2. **Always ask for a twin discount.** From baby stores to music classes, it never hurts to ask.
3. **Accept hand-me-downs and gifts.** Say yes if they are needed.
4. **You don't need two of everything.** Think about ways to make do with one.
5. **Avoid impulse and reaction buys.** One mom said she forces herself to answer the question "Do we really need this?" at checkout when buying things for her twins.

Go generic. For many moms, brand is an important factor in choosing formula, bottles, and more. We strive to make our babies as comfortable as possible. But with other things, such as diapers and wipes, you might want to shop generic, like our survey moms, as a major money-saving tactic.

Clip coupons. Even if you never considered coupons worth the effort before, the expense associated with raising twins might change your mind. Toys R Us/Babies R Us mails coupon books and also frequently provides in-store circulars. And, in the spirit of double everything, you can double up with coupons, too. For example, one mom we surveyed suggests getting a Babies R Us diaper coupon and using it in conjunction with a Huggies coupon for twice the savings. You can even put out the word to family, as Christina did; her sister-in-law would frequently mail a batch.

Join the clubs. Several grocery and drugstore chains offer money back if you join their in-store clubs. No fee is required, but you will need to carry your membership card to access your savings. CVS, a drugstore chain, literally gives you coupons with dollar values (and expiration dates) that can be used to buy anything in the store.

The bottom line, according to Gugle, "Determine a family budget, then live within your means."

BREAK IT DOWN

To help you take that first step toward making a realistic budget, here's an overview of expenses you can count on and some strategies for savings.

EXPENSE	USAGE	SAVINGS
No avoiding		
Diapers	• Two three-month-olds can go through a dozen diapers daily.	• 1800diapers.com • Diaper clubs like Pampers' Grow with Me • Coupons
Formula/Food	• Two three-month-olds will eat upward of 36 ounces daily. • Two one-year-olds eat at least three meals a day.	• eBay • Warehouse clubs (but be mindful of expiration dates). • Homemade baby purees are a cheaper alternative to jars, and they can be worked in with meals for the rest of the family.

EXPENSE	USAGE	SAVINGS
Car seats	• Must have two infant bucket seats; babies stay in them generally six months; after 20 lbs., they move on to seats they can stay in for years (typically until about 40 lbs.).	• Limited usage means fellow moms (even two different friends of singletons) could loan you theirs; sometimes the less popular prints or colors can be bought on sale.
Baby care (soap, shampoo, hygiene)	• If you bathe your twins every day, you can easily go through a 28-ounce bottle of shampoo in a month.	• Load up at the hospital with gifts from Johnson's for new moms; combination hair and body cleanser can help; warehouse clubs sell oversize bottles, and they never expire!
Stroller	• You might need a Snap 'N Go to carry the two-bucket car seats; or buy a stroller that can convert from infants to kids (like the favorite of Cathy and many survey moms, Urban Mountain Buggy).	• Gently used is fine; even friends with older, staggered singletons can hand those down or loan them to you.
At your discretion		
Clothing	• Of course, clothing is required, but you can manage on less than you think.	• Hand-me-downs • Tag sales • Use credit card points for gift certificates at baby-Gap. • Shop at the outlets. • Buy a size or two ahead at sale time instead of full price in season.

EXPENSE	USAGE	SAVINGS
Gear (bouncy seats, ExerSaucers, etc.)	• Infants need the most equipment—bouncy seats, swings, and transportation devices of all kinds. • Toddlers need a stroller most of all.	• Perfect hand-me-downs, especially since your need for these will be temporary; try to tap into parents whose kids are leaving the baby stage; they will be thrilled to hand these off to you! Go for two different families if you have to, nothing needs to match.
Restaurants	• Children might start ordering from the menu around one year.	• Some places offer family discounts. For example, kids eat free before 6:00 P.M. at IHOP. We try to order one meal for our twins, then a side of veggies to share.
Classes/Activities	• Mommy and Me classes can start at six months of age.	• Some classes can run upward of $300 per student per session; libraries are usually free; seek out town or city-run programs that are typically offered at more affordable rates. If you need to bring a helper, you might need to factor in babysitting costs, too.
Toys	• Twins don't need two of everything; rotating play stations at a young age can help them get used to taking turns.	• We learned after having our first singleton children that parents can definitely get away with not buying their children any toys at all—between grandparents and other well-wishers, they seem to get more than they need.

Money Relief: The Days You'll Rejoice to Be Moving On

- Switching from formula to regular milk
- Getting out of diapers and Pull-Ups and into underwear
- Selling your cribs, stroller, high chairs, and safety gates
- The day the twins enter the public school system
- When you can hire a high schooler to babysit at night instead of a high-cost adult

BIG-TICKET ITEMS

Some of the larger expenses associated with raising twins require more strategy than clipping coupons from the weekend paper. We've made a list of the most common big-ticket items and given you an idea of the cost associated with each, so you can begin working these expenses into your budget.

Baby nurse. More than 30 percent of the moms we surveyed said they hired a baby nurse to help care for their newborn twins. Absent some nearby, willing, and exceptionally capable family members, considering professional help is common for new moms of twins. Fees begin around $250 per night (typically defined as a twelve-hour period) and can go up to $1,800 per week (round-the-clock care for six days and nights). You need not become a full-time employer—there are nurses who can be hired a few nights a week. Check out our "Good Help" chapter, page 169, for more about the different types of help you might need and how much it all costs.

Child care. The general consensus among moms we surveyed is that they ended up hiring *way more* help than they had anticipated. Cathy's family hired an au pair (a relatively inexpensive, full-time, child care option) for a year because they decided it would ultimately be cheaper than the amount of à la carte babysitting, paid at a fixed price per hour, that they felt they needed. Even if you don't hire a steady part- or full-time sitter, you should expect to pay up for nights you do hire someone to watch the twins. Some sitters charge a little extra for multiple children, regardless of the workload (for example, even if the twins are sleeping the whole time the sitter is there).

Some of the moms we surveyed suggest sharing babysitting with sisters, friends, and neighbors; the rationale is that if you are going to have to pay up for more than one child anyway, why not add one or two more and then split the cost? Others (like Christina) use mother's helpers as a less expensive alternative to adult care for the times when they just need an extra set of hands or someone willing to engage in some hard-core playtime. You might need to stick around more with a young person, but it should be cheaper than hiring a grown-up.

Education. Parents of twins should carefully consider two preschool tuitions and hefty fees for activities such as music and art classes. The main point of preschool and toddler classes is to engage your children and promote social interaction with others. That can also be accomplished in free or inexpensive settings such as play groups at your home or classes at the pubic library. Or try to limit yourself to enrolling in one activity with the twins per season. During the winter months, when one or both of your twins might battle frequent colds or other illnesses, consider taking a break from all things structured because there is nothing worse

College Planning—Oh My!

We are all looking at two children going through four years of college AT THE EXACT SAME TIME! College planning is the biggest expense most parents face, but starting early and saving consistently makes all the difference. Gugle urges us, "Don't wait. If you lose those early years, you lose that opportunity to put money away." The best vehicle available today is a 529 college savings plan that allows you to save money tax-free, up to $250,000 total per child. Each state has its own plan with assets managed by independent investment management firms. You are not limited to investing in *your* state's plan, but sometimes there are tax advantages to consider with the plan of the state you live in. Check out savingforcollege.com to learn more about 529 plans and for a calculator that helps you break down monthly savings rates based on the age of your children. No customized version for twins is available, so you'll need to save at twice the rate shown. The good news is that these are regular mutual fund accounts, so most allow contributions of as little as $25—perfect for holiday and birthday gift checks.

Another education savings option is the Coverdell account because you can use the money for any educational expense, not just college (529 plans are for college only). For example, if you want to send your children to private elementary school, you can save up to $2,000 per year in a Coverdell account. If this is something you think you might consider, you can make annual contributions while your twins are young and let the investment grow tax-free until middle or high school, or even college. Savingforcollege.com is a great resource for Coverdell accounts, too.

than ponying up the class fee and then missing most of the classes. And check with your employer to see if you can contribute pre-tax dollars to a Dependent Care Reimbursement Account for daycare or preschool tuition costs.

Housing. Many moms report that they instantly felt like they did not have enough house to accommodate their twin babies and all of their stuff, even if the twins share a room. Gugle cautions parents of twins against taking on more mortgage or rent than you can comfortably handle. "Getting in over your head means monthly debt that can quickly spiral out of your control," he warns. He adds that moving, in and of itself, is not a cheap endeavor. Rather than feel the squeeze in your current space, he suggests you clear out clutter and get organized to make the most of your place and look for ways to add on to your current house. Think long and hard to justify whether or not your family really needs more space. If you simply must move, consider buying more house in a less expensive neighborhood. He also cautions, "If you are going to buy a new home, don't be tempted by 'introductory' mortgage specials that can explode later and bust the budget, just to get into a house (for example, negatively amortizing mortgages)."

Recreation. Vacations for large families (and you qualify simply by having twins) might be best in all-inclusive places such as Beaches or Club Med. Many of these are very family friendly and you'll know the complete cost of your package from the outset, as hidden or surprising costs are typically minimal. Or consider renting a house or condo and doing your own grocery shopping (outside the resort area is probably best). We know some families who take time off work and stay home with the kids to enjoy local attractions.

Budgeting for twins can mean making adjustments for special items such as eating out. Instead of a single $6.95 kids' meal, you

The Seasonal Spending Factor

When planning your budget, you'll want to be mindful of annual spending cycles. For example, back-to-school time often calls for new backpacks, shoes, activity fees, sports gear, and more. The winter season may mean holiday gifts, new boots, jackets, snow pants, ski rentals, ice skates, helmets, and more. The summer season may be kinder to your wallet—flip-flops are usually pretty cheap!

Retirement Savings? What's That?

A basic tenet of parenting is that as parents, we tend to put our needs behind those of our children. Financially, this means that things such as retirement planning contributions take a backseat to car seats, double strollers, and other twin-related expenses. But as Gugle reminds us, there is no scholarship for retirement. If you are not taking care of your own retirement funding, you won't have it when you need it. He suggests doing what you can whether it be by contributing monthly to your company's 401(k) plan or making annual tax-free contributions to an IRA or Roth IRA. Check out motleyfool.com for more information about retirement planning.

are paying $13.90 with no guarantee your twins will even eat the food. Sometimes we think twice about stopping for ice cream when it's a $4 expense instead of $2 and if we already have ice pops in the freezer at home.

IN CASE OF EMERGENCY

As a parent of twins, you know better than anyone that it takes a lot of energy and resources to care for your children. And even though no one wants to think about the worst happening, with twins, the repercussions of not dealing with plans for your children can be great. Gugle knows it's not a pleasant subject to think about, but he suggests that both you and your spouse consider taking on enough life insurance to cover larger future liabilities such as paying off your home and covering education costs. Both working and nonworking spouses need to carry an adequate amount. He says, "I've seen folks who don't cover the nonworking spouse. If something happened to the parent who stays home with the twins, the surviving spouse's life would be thrown into turmoil and that might affect their career. I encourage people to consider more than simply replacement income."

He also suggests affordable term life insurance when you're younger because you're buying pure insurance, dollar for dollar. To calculate what you need, tabulate what it's going to cost to put your kids through college, pay off the mortgage for the surviving spouse, secure adequate cash flow, and cover child care costs so the surviving spouse can work.

Another important issue to consider is estate planning. For parents, this involves establishing guardianship. If something were to happen to you and your husband, who would be responsible for caring for and bringing up your children? It's a tough decision to make, because not everyone on either side of your family could handle the mammoth responsibility of raising your twins. Gugle suggests talking to an estate planning attorney to establish durable and health care powers of attorney. These name decision makers to act in your place should you be critically injured and put official documents in place so things are not left to the courts to determine. Gugle encourages you to talk to the people you plan to name in order to ensure that they agree to cover for you if need be. Also, once you get all of these important documents signed, sealed, and delivered, store them somewhere at home where the twins won't find them (for fear that they will color them, cut them into confetti, or spill something on them).

Twincidentals: Protecting Your Relationship

Many, many couples, even happy ones, fight over money. It is a stressful issue. Having twins can also be tough on a relationship because of the time, energy, and emotional demands. Put the two together and even the most solid relationship is going to take a hit. We suggest trying to minimize the pressure in advance as much as possible. Make sure you agree on what's required and what's helpful when spending money on your twins. For example, good help is great and necessary, but it can also be expensive. If your partner does not bear the brunt of the child care, he or she might not realize how difficult it is to do without an extra set of hands. One way to take some of the burden off you, your partner, and the relationship is to hire a professional financial adviser. Gugle is a fee-only planner, meaning that his compensation is non-commission driven. Check out fpanet.org or napfa.org to learn more.

Sadly, one of the biggest money-savers for us moms of twins is the absence of a social life with our partners. Once the twins arrive, between their care and your lack of sleep, it's hard to muster the energy to get dressed and go out to dinner with your partner. Tack on the financial savings and suddenly it makes sense to stay home night after night. While this is a viable and sometimes necessary short-term solution, we urge you to take steps to avoid making it a long-term solution. Cathy and her husband have downgraded their restaurant choices, so they'll go out for burgers instead of fancy meals to offset the babysitting costs associated with the night out. Christina and her husband established regular Friday night at-home dates. They try to cook a nice meal, set the table, and wear clean clothes to cuddle up and watch the latest Netflix shipment. The point is to get dressed, sit at a table for two, and actually talk. It's amazing how one night of laughing and talking together can rekindle your connection and get you through weeks of stressful parenting. Your life might be on hold, but it's not over. Do what you can to fit your pre-twins life into your budget; it's an investment in your future.

TWINESSENTIALS

Every mom wants to know what she needs to get for her new baby, and for moms of twins, that pressure is magnified. Here is our twin spin on products and resources to help you make good decisions for your multiples.

The Top 5 Survey Standouts

The double stroller (start with a double Snap 'N Go, then upgrade to a Maclaren or Urban Mountain Buggy when the twins are about four months).

A good nursing pillow like the E-Z 2-Nurse twins pillow.

Two indoor baby swings (Fisher-Price cradle swings were mentioned. Cathy and Christina never used these, much to the shock of our friend with two sets of twins. Instead, we were fans of bouncy seats, play mats, and Exer-Saucers).

Two Boppy pillows (for bottle-feeding and play time).

Bottle helpers (Although not recommended by pediatricians, our moms liked the Little Wonders Bottle Proper from greatbabyproducts.com and the Bottle Bundle Bottle Prop. Survey moms also praised the Podee self-feeding bottles, which are easy for young babies to hold and drink from without much help from Mom.)

Where Moms of Twins Shop for Baby Stuff

The Warehouse Clubs (Costco, Sam's Club, BJ's)

The MOM's Tag Sale

Target

WalMart

Toys R Us or Babies R Us

Buy Buy Baby

Gymboree

Tiny Love

Greatbabyproducts.com

babyGap

Crewcuts

Lands' End

L. L. Bean

Books Moms of Twins Love

When You're Expecting Twins, Triplets, or Quads: Proven Guidelines for a Healthy Multiple Pregnancy by Dr. Barbara Luke and Tamara Eberline

Having Twins: A Parent's Guide to Multiple Pregnancy, Birth, and Early Childhood by Elizabeth Noble

On Becoming Babywise by Gary Ezzo and Robert Bucknam

Secrets of the Baby Whisperer by Tracy Hogg

Healthy Sleep Habits, Happy Child by Marc Weissbluth, M.D.

What to Expect When You're Expecting (4th edition) by Heidi Murkoff and Sharon Mazel

Girlfriends' Guide to Pregnancy by Vicki Lovine

Your Pregnancy Week by Week (5th edition) by Glade B. Curtis and Judith Schuler

Ready or Not Here We Come by Elizabeth Lyons

The Multiples Manual by Lynn Lorenz and Shelley Dieterichs

The Baby Book by William Sears, M.D., and Martha Sears, R.N.

The Nursing Mother's Companion by Kathleen Huggins, R.N., M.S.

Baby Bargains (7th edition) by Denise Fields

Siblings Without Rivalry by Adele Faber and Elaine Mazlish

Web sites Moms of Multiples Love

Nomotc.org (The National Organization of Mothers of Twins Clubs)

Twinsetmoms.com (shameless plug from us!)

sidelines.org (for pregnant moms on bed rest)

IVFconnections.com (for pregnant moms on bed rest)

dona.org (for doula information)

lllusa.org (for lactation consultant information)

multiplebirthfamilies.com

breastfeeding.com

Twinslaw.com (for updates on states and school separation policies)

Babycenter.com

Babytalk.com

Parenting.com

tripletconnection.org (for moms of triplets)

Magazines Moms of Twins Love

Babytalk

Parenting

Parents

Cookie

Twins magazine

NOMOTC Notebook

People

InStyle

Things to Make Pregnant Moms of Multiples More Comfy

Maternity belt (amazon.com or fitmaternity.com)
Body-size pillow (The Company Store catalogue)
Preggie Pops or Preggie Pop Drops (threelollies.com)
B-natal Green Apple Lozenges or B-natal Cherry-Flavored
TheraPops (ladytobaby.com)

Stuff to Get Preemie Twins

NICU T-shirts (for babies under 2 pounds)
"Weight sized" preemie clothes (for babies over 2 pounds or
    30 weeks' gestation): cotton hats, NICU T-shirts, NICU bag
    sleepers, and socks
Supplies for each preemie twin at home: preemie bag sleepers,
    preemie onesies, preemie footies, preemie hats, and preemie
    socks
Several bottles of hand sanitizer
Hospital-grade breast pump (you can rent one to take home)
Medical-grade scale (use it to weigh your babies at home)

Where Moms of Preemie Twins Shop

gap.com
ittybittybundles.com
preemiesrus.com
preemie.com
snuggletown.com
preemie-yums.com
jacquispreemiepride.com
preemietees.com

What Moms of Preemie Twins Can Read for Help

Preemies: The Essential Guide for Parents of Premature Babies by Dana Wechsler Linden, Emma Trenti Paroli, and Mia Wechsler Doron, M.D.

Special Report: Premature Twins and Triplets by *Twins* magazine

Preemie magazine

Where Moms of Preemies Can Surf for Info and Support

Marchofdimes.org (a national nonprofit dedicated to prematurity awareness)

ttmf.org (The Tiny Miracles Foundation, a nonprofit group in Connecticut devoted to supporting parents of premature infants)

twinsmagazine.com (visit the Twins Mall)

CarePages.com (a free online service that helps you stay in touch with family and friends)

birth23.org (a national service to help parents secure speech, physical, and occupational therapy for developmentally delayed young children)

What New Moms of Twins Can Wear to Look Hot

Helpful undergarments (push-up bras, camisoles with built-in bras, postpartum wrap belts, and lower-body girdles found at Target and GapBody)

Belly-hiding, above-the-knee A-line or bubble dresses in structured fabrics (like linen and wool)

Maternity jeans (by Juicy and Seven for All Mankind)

Wrap dresses to flaunt bust and play down hips

Where New Moms of Twins Shop for Transition Wardrobes

Gap

Old Navy

H & M

Zara

Target

J. Crew

Discount stores (Loehmann's, Marshalls, T.J. Maxx)

eBay (for shoes if your feet grew during pregnancy)

Stuff to Get Organized

Wallet-size coupon organizer

Daily planner (momAgenda.com has room for your twins on it)

Large white board

Itzbeen (to keep track of twins' feedings, poops, naps, and more)

StrollAway—an over-the-door stroller storage system strong
enough to hold a double stroller to free up space in your home.
Check out metrotots.com to learn more.

EAT

Stuff for Breast-feeding Twins

A good, comfy nursing pillow for twins. Try the E-Z 2-Nurse
twins pillow (doubleblessings.com or justmultiples.com) or My
Breast Friend

A strong double pump (try renting one from your hospital or
check out one from Medela), or you can try wearing a pump bra
(we were surprised by this one!)

A bedside cooler with an ice pack or a mini-fridge to store just-
pumped milk

Stuff for Bottle-feeding Infant Twins

Only get a couple of bottles from a couple different brands at first, because each twin may have his or her own preference. After your twins get comfortable with a bottle, then you can buy a total of eight or so bottles each. (Some survey moms swear by Dr. Brown's bottles for gassy babies.)

Podee self-feeding bottles (a big hit with survey moms)

A place for the twins to safely recline: either two bouncy chairs, two car-seat buckets, the double stroller (a side-by-side makes bottle-feeding easier), or two Boppies

Stuff for Feeding Twins Solid Foods

A place for the twins to sit up: either two traditional high chairs (Eddie Bauer and Safety 1st make wooden chairs with three-point harnesses that are easy to clean; Peg Perego's Prima Pappa is an easy-clean plastic chair with tray inserts that fit on the removable top); two portable high chairs (that use belts to fasten on safely to household seats); or a side-by-side double stroller

Bowls, cups, and utensils: moms with identical twins like to color-code these, and other moms of twins like to get all the same color or character to avoid twin fights down the road

Bibs (look for ones that twins can't easily rip off or that have a pocket at the bottom to help you catch double messes)

POOP

Stuff to Diaper-change Twins

A week's worth of diapers (at first, each twin goes through about 10 diapers a day, so that's about 140 diapers in a week)
A package of diapers in the next size

Tons of wipes (we each still keep an extra big box with more than 700 wipes in our homes)

Where Moms of Twins Get Diapers

1800diapers.com
Pampers.com
Huggies.com
diapernet.com
gdiapers.com
Whole Foods and other natural retailers
Warehouse clubs (Costco, BJ's, and Sam's Club)

Stuff to Potty-train Twins

Undies (consider that you have to sort their undies in the laundry, so make it easier on yourself and get them all the same or in one distinct color or pattern for each twin)

Portable potty or toilet-seat insert (you may only need to start with one of these if only one twin is ready to learn)

SLEEP

Stuff for Newborn and Infant Twins

Places to nap (two-bucket car seats, two bouncy seats, a Moses basket, a bassinet, a Pack 'n Play, indoor baby swings, or a crib)

Places for longer stretches of sleep together (one crib, one bassinet, one Pack 'n Play)

Places for longer stretches of sleep by themselves (two cribs, two bassinets, two Pack 'n Plays)

Swaddling blankets (miracleblanket.com, LovingBabyInc.com, halosleep.com, kiddopotamus.com)

Stuff for Toddler Twins

Room-darkening shades

Crib tents (to keep toddlers from escaping, available at onestepahead.com or leapsandbounds.com)

Two toddler beds or two big-kid beds (with rails, so twins don't fall out)

BATHE

Stuff to Clean Newborn or Infant Twins

Washcloths (have at least fouteen in stock) and a gentle cleanser (sponge baths are less taxing than real baths, so stick with these for a few weeks)

A bathing spot for one twin at a time (moms of multiples use the kitchen sink if it's deep enough and has a handheld faucet; or they use an infant bathtub)

Stuff to Clean Twins Six Months and Up

A bathing spot for one at a time (a tub-ring seat may help your baby sit up with more stability) or a bathing spot for two at a time (two tub-ring seats or a tub liner)

Stuff to Make Bathing Safer

Non-skid bathtub stickers
Slip-proof bath mat
One spout guard

Stuff to Clean Toddler Twins

One kiddie pool (to put in a large shower or to use as an outdoor tub in warm weather) or an outdoor shower (seasonally available at Home Depot, Costco, or in the *Frontgate* catalogue)

PLAY

Stuff for Infant Twins

Rotating play stations (moms of multiples like to feed and change twins, then have them play for a while before they take a nap. To keep twins safe and busy, consider getting a couple of these options for your play stations: a bouncy seat, a jumperoo, a portable swing, an ExerSaucer, a play mat, or a play yard with soft toys)

Stuff for Crawlers and Walkers

Gates to confine twins' play to one baby-proofed room, to protect them from trouble on the stairs and to keep them out of dangerous rooms

Where to Surf for Babyproofing Supplies and Safety Tips

Onestepahead.com or leapsandbounds.com
Home Depot
usfa.gov or sparky.org. (for fire safety info)

HELP

Where Moms of Twins Surf for Child Care Info

NCCIC.org (National Child care Information Center)

Childaware.org (for tips on finding good care)

gentlehandschildcare.com

sittercity.com, craigslist.com, eNannySource.com, nannypoppins.com (for ideas on caregivers' costs and qualifications)

babysafeamerica.com, babysitters.com, crimcheck.com, integctr.com, findoutnow.net, or nannybackgrounds.com (for information on conducting interviews and background checks)

redcross.org (to learn about babysitter and CPR classes)

mollymaid.com or merrymaid.com (for ideas on how much a cleaning service can cost and what they can do for you)

ACKNOWLEDGMENTS

We are so grateful to all of the moms of multiples across the country who participated in our survey. They lend the book credence, context, and a great foundation. These moms gave so generously of their time telling their twin war stories, sharing the amazing things they witness every day as moms of twins, and readily offering their most successful secrets and strategies.

We're also lucky to have found so many parents of twins with professional expertise—from personal styling to pediatrics—who were gracious enough to reveal their unique work and home perspectives. Check out pages xi–xii for the details on our panel of experts.

We especially want to thank our wise and gracious agent, Susan Ginsburg, and our lovely and patient editor, Lindsay Orman. We are grateful to all of the wonderful people at Three Rivers Press and Crown who embraced our idea and us—Philip Patrick, Carrie Thornton, Linda Kaplan, Julie Kraut, Annsley Rosner, and Sarah Breivogel.

Along the way, we were touched by the willingness of so many to help move us up the learning curve—Annie Mackenzie, Rob Mackenzie, Edward J. Boyle, Edward P. Boyle, Susan Kane, Patty Onderko, Jamie Reidy, Kathleen Millard, Susan Swimmer, Bari Nan Cohen, Amy Newman, Leeann Leahy, Pam Fahey, Rob

Densen, Brian Pearlman, Selina Cicogna, John Dubaz, M.D., everyone at The Tiny Miracles Foundation, the dads from our focus group, and the moms in our local MOMs club. We're also indebted to Kristin Vrooman, Christi Hanson, Kara Guthrie, Ashley Dineen, Annie Sullivan, and Brigid Maguire. And we're extremely appreciative of our interns—Chrissy DeMarzo and Haley Cook.

We are most grateful to our families and friends for their support.

Cathy thanks Rick, Luke, Will, Jack, and Emmet for daily inspiration. Christina thanks her thoughtful and helpful husband and her three adorable nonskootchy kids.

INDEX

ABOUT THE AUTHORS

Christina Boyle currently works at home as a contributing editor to *Babytalk*. She has also been a senior editor at *YM* and *Redbook* and executive editor of *Modern Bride,* and her work has appeared in *Cosmopolitan, Good Housekeeping, Shape, Fitness,* and *Ladies' Home Journal.* Christina and her husband have one singleton daughter and boy/girl twins.

Cathleen Stahl is currently vice president at Allianz Global Investors, a leading asset management firm. Previously, she served as senior consultant at the advocacy marketing firm Tiller LLC and as vice president of business development in the Wealth Management group at OppenheimerFunds. During her tenure there, she also managed the firm's high-profile Women & Investing program. Cathy and her husband have two singleton sons and fraternal boy twins.

Both Twin Set Moms live in Connecticut.

Premature birth is a challenge many families with multiples face. That's why Tiny Miracles and March of Dimes are very important to us. We encourage you to learn more about premature birth and these two organizations and consider supporting the amazing work that they do.

Tiny Miracles
ttmf.org

March of Dimes
marchofdimes.com